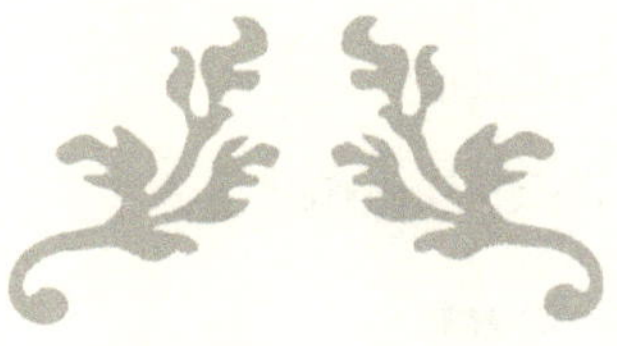

VOY -001 CRUISING WITH THE LEAD NURSE

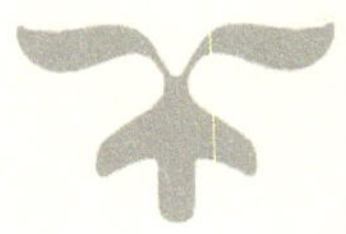

Aslam Goolam Hoosen

Table of Contents

Chapter One: Home Port

Leana Ria, a seasoned cruise ship nurse with 15 years' experience and twelve of those as Lead nurse. A knot of excitement and anxiety twisted in her stomach as she awoke on July 25th, 2014, the day she would finally board the Majestic Voyager, the result of her tireless efforts. The alarm clock displayed 6:45 am, its red digits seeming to mock her with their steady tick, urging her to get ready for the breakfast buffet and catch the crew shuttle. 'Fresh slate,' she whispered to the empty room, the words meant to reassure but instead felt like a hollow promise. Blinking away sleep, she swung her legs off the bed, her mind already racing with questions: Could she effectively lead this diverse team? There are always personality clashes, incompetent staff, and the responsibility of running a medical centre, ensuring adequate stock levels and maintaining emergency equipment.

. A swift wash-up later, she slipped into her everyday uniform, pride swelling at its crisp lines. She hefted her luggage and rode the elevator down, the hum a quiet prelude to the day's roar.

The scent of coffee drew Leana into the busy breakfast buffet where she quickly assembled a plate of eggs, bacon, and toast before retreating to a secluded spot to dine. As she surveyed the room, her heart raced at the sight of familiar crewmates from her fifteen-year career: a Peruvian deckhand she'd worked with on the Caribbean Voyager and a Ukrainian chef who'd shared a midnight coffee during a Pacific storm. Their presence was comforting yet transient; she smiled at them, receiving warm smiles and nods in return. The buffet was a vibrant tapestry of humanity, with seafarers from India, the Philippines, Peru, Ukraine, Romania, Indonesia, and Italy—all part of the beautiful melting pot that Leana was honoured to be part of.

As she sipped her coffee, she mulled over the day ahead. She would collaborate with a diverse medical team, including two doctors and three nurses and a healthcare administrator from various countries. The challenge of leading such a group both excited and daunted her, but she knew her experience and dedication would guide her through any obstacles.

The shuttle screeched to a halt in front of the hotel entrance and a burly driver with a thick beard and red cap emerged. "All crew for the Majestic Voyager," he bellowed, "grab your luggage and meet me at the shuttle!"

Leana eagerly gathered her luggage and followed her crewmates to the vehicle. The driver carefully stowed their belongings in the back to make sure there was enough space for everyone.

As they drove towards New York Harbour, Leana's excitement grew as she imagined her new home for the next four months: the grand Majestic Voyager cruise ship. The shuttle moved closer to Downtown Manhattan; Leana gasped in awe as she caught a glimpse of the Majestic Voyager. This magnificent 110,000-tonne cruise ship dwarfed everything else in sight, radiating an air of opulence worthy of royalty. Rumours of its size and grandeur had not done it justice—she was in utter disbelief at the sheer magnitude of this majestic vessel with its glimmering towers and luxurious balconies that reached out into the vast expanse of the sky. As she admired the elegance of the ship, she felt her anticipation grow to soar on board, alongside 3,200 passengers and 1,000 crew on their own voyage of discovery, ready to explore a never-ending array of delectable dining and exhilarating entertainment.

The shuttle pulled into the Manhattan Cruise Terminal, and Leana's eyes stretched wide at the ship's towering bulk. Crew swarmed the docks, prepping for the seven-day haul, a machine humming in sync. Stepping onto the port, she drew a sharp breath, steeling herself for the lead nurse weight settling on her shoulders.

Luggage in tow, the crew neared the gangway where a sharp-dressed team waited—navy uniforms crisp, gold buttons glinting under the sun. A woman, late forties, anchored the group, her gaze slicing through them before she spoke.

"Welcome aboard, everyone!" declared Melissa Cleaver, her tone immediately commanding attention.

Having served as HR director for several years aboard various vessels, she had developed a reputation for efficiency and a no-nonsense approach. Her age, around late forties, was evident from the fine lines around her eyes and mouth, yet there was a youthful energy about her, suggesting she still found joy in her work. "Apologies for the slight delay with the boarding process; it seems things are moving a little slower than usual today," she explained briskly, though her smile indicated she wasn't too concerned.

"In the meantime, my colleagues and I are here to assist, ensuring all necessary documentation is completed so you can officially join our team here on the Majestic Voyager, a truly remarkable vessel." As she spoke, she gestured towards two assistants standing nearby: Eleanor, known for her meticulous attention to detail when it came to administrative tasks, and Ravi, who always seemed to remain calm and collected even in the most hectic situations. Together, they formed a solid support system, helping new hires and returning crew feel welcome and integrated swiftly.

"Once your paperwork's done, Rebello's got vessel safety and familiarization lined up." She stretched out a hand, gathering passports, medical docs, seaman's books, crisis training certs—the works.

The crew buzzed with purpose, professionalism laced with warmth—smiles flashed, chatter rippled between them. Leana passed her stack to Melissa, who rifled through it, quick and sure.

"All clear," Melissa said, grinning. "Safety trainings in the conference room—everything you need's there. Looking forward to working with you, Leana."

"You too," Leana replied, mirroring her smile.

Striding through the ship, Leana felt excitement and unease wrestling in her chest, same as dawn. She reached the crew conference room, greeted by Emilio Rebello, the training manager—a live wire welcoming newbies and vets alike. He rolled out the training officer, Mario Vincenzo, an Italian in a white uniform, three stripes gleaming on his shoulders.

Mario's hands danced as he spoke. "Never cross a watertight door mid-motion!" he barked, jabbing a finger for emphasis.

Mario explained what to do in the event of a fire, listed the emergency phone numbers, and demonstrated the cruise ship's alarms. The first demonstration was the 'man overboard' alarm: two loud blasts of the ship horn followed by a voice over the intercom announcing, "Man overboard plus location."

The other announcements included fire, pollution and damage to the ship. Out of nowhere, the training officer called on Leana and asked, "Can you tell us about the announcement for medical emergencies?"

Although Leana was caught off guard, she was familiar with all the announcements. She stood up and smiled.

"Code Blue team, Code Blue team, and the location of the incident."

"Thanks, Lead Nurse," Mario said before moving on to discuss passenger and crew muster stations. He demonstrated how to don a lifejacket and where to find extras during an emergency. The focus of the Vessel Safety Familiarisation Training was the safety and security of the crew and guests.

Next was the environmental officer, Bruno Rodriguez from Panama; he spoke about taking care of the ocean and making sure that no items flew into the sea. He also stressed the importance of waste segregation of food and materials like glass, cans, batteries, razors, so on. Finally, he concluded his training on chemical management: namely how to manage spills and to only use designated chemicals approved by the company.

Lastly, was the chief of security, Rajesh Singh, and he stressed that it was every crew member's responsibility to mind the safety and security of the ship.

The crew was then taken on a tour of the ship and shown how to operate the watertight and splash tight doors if necessary, during an emergency. On their way to the passenger muster station, Leana and the other crew members gasped as they entered the guest area of the atrium. Before them, Queen Eleanor the Graceful stared out from a mural that almost seemed to hum with the power of its subject. The emerald and lace of Eleanor's sweeping gown cascaded to the floor like a great waterfall. The pearls draped around her neck and bodice caught the light as if to capture the stars for all eternity. Her eyes were deep and glittering: a wellspring of wisdom gathered through decades of ruling her kingdom with grace, dignity and peace.

This was the heart of the Majestic Voyager, Eleanor's Court Deck centres on the Eleanor Atrium, a resplendent three-story nexus of crystal elevators, polished marble floors, and gilded flourishes. It houses guest relations, port excursion counters, and the lower tier of the Queen's Hall Dining Room, an opulent venue adorned with sparkling chandeliers and claret velvet curtains.

Once the crew pinned down every muster station for emergencies, training wrapped. Leana headed to the medical centre, pulse up, ready to face her new crew.

The medical centre thrummed as stock rolled in, staff weaving through prep for the voyage. Leana watched, sizing up the bustle.

"Leana!" a voice cut through, yanking her focus. She spun to find Dr. Alberto Gutierrez, senior doc from Mexico, her boss, weaving through Deck 0's hallway crowd. His thick accent and broad grin eased her nerves. "Good to see you again," he said, gripping her hand firm. Leana worked with Dr Gutierrez on the Caribbean Voyager a few years back, and they have developed a trusted relationship, which is always essential when the head of the department and the lead nurse share the same goal.

"Same, Dr. Gutierrez," she shot back, matching his smile. "Ready to roll with you."

"Perfect," he said, waving the crew closer. "Meet your team: Dr. Abhishek Srinivas, nurses Rodrigo, Mkhwanazi, Jit, and Roberta, our admin. Team, tell Lead Nurse Leana about yourselves—where you're from, how long you've sailed."

A nurse stood in front of Leana, smiling. She had a soft face and a kindly look, with wide, compassionate brown eyes that sparkled like two warm-hued gems. She was small and chubby, with short curly hair that bounced around her shoulders when she moved. "Hi, I am Mkhwanazi!" she said quickly, throwing her hand out in a wave. "I am from Johannesburg, South Africa. I have been working on cruise ships for two years. It is nice to meet you."

"Hello, I'm Dr. Srinivas from Kerala, India. Nice to meet you," he said, his voice warm but his face unsmiling. He was in his early thirties, with deep brown skin, short hair, and a dusting of facial hair over an average build.

Leana turned, feeling a sharp, icy gaze cut through the room. An older woman stepped forward, her movements precise but tense, and extended a hand. 'Nurse Jit,' she said, her voice clipped and cool, carrying the weight of twelve years at sea. Her angular face, framed by shoulder-length hair tied back in a tight ponytail, revealed greying temples and eyes hinting at a history of battles—both medical and personal. In her late fifties, she stood with arms crossed, her expression a fortress, with no trace of a smile. Leana sensed her displeasure immediately and wondered if it stemmed from professional rivalry, exhaustion, or a deeper wound from decades at sea.

The last nurse smiled warmly. "Hello, Leana!" he said in an upbeat voice. "My name is Rodrigo, and I'm from the Philippines. This is my last trip before I take some time off. Five years of working on cruises, you know!"

He seemed relaxed, but his eyes were heavy with exhaustion, like he was nursing a hangover. Despite his age—he couldn't have been older than his late twenties—he appeared to be enjoying life on the ship.

Roberta Munoz was a tall, light-skinned woman with long black hair, dark eyes and smooth, striking features. She strode up to Leana like she owned the world and said, "Greetings, I'm Roberta Munoz from Brazil. I adore globetrotting and staying in shape. I'm new here and still learning—it's exciting to acquire different abilities." Her voice was commanding but not harsh and carried the elocution of someone who spoke often before large crowds.

Leana found her words soothing. "I love your hair; I wish mine were the same! And you could be my personal trainer!"

Roberta laughed and responded, "If you teach me everything I need to learn, then I'll pass on all my knowledge to you."

Then it was Leana's turn to introduce herself. "Thanks, all. I'm Leana Ria, Cape Town, South Africa—fifteen years on ships, twelve as lead nurse." Her eyes flicked to Nurse Jit, sharp and steady, a quiet claim staked in the pause.

With the introductions done, they all moved towards the nurses' station. Leana could not help but marvel at the diverse group she would be working with. She knew that navigating cultural differences could sometimes be tricky, but she was confident that their shared passion for helping others would bridge any gaps.

"Alright, team," Leana began, taking charge as the lead nurse of the Majestic Voyager. "Remember, communication is key. Let's make sure we're all on the same page throughout this voyage."

"Message received," Rodrigo said firmly, his voice reassuring.

The others nodded in agreement, their expressions determined. Leana settled into her spot at the nurses' station and the phone began to shrill – a call to the emergency line.

Jit snatched the phone, voice tight. A woman's sobs crackled through, frantic—her husband collapsed outside Deck 6 elevator in the lobby.

"Which one, ma'am? Front, mid, back?" Jit ground out, teeth clenched.

Stammering tears spilled back. "Uh… near cabin 6214!"

Leana's eyes hit the station map, pinning cabin 6214 near the front elevator. She turned, barking, "Team, huddle up—collapse, Deck 6 forward. Jit, with me. Rodrigo, Mkhwanazi, standby for backup. Dr. Gutierrez, you set?"

"Ready when you need me," Dr. Gutierrez nodded, steady.

"Move," Leana snapped, slinging an emergency bag over her shoulder, Jit grabbing the oxygen tank. She lunged for the door, then froze—Mkhwanazi's shout cutting through.

"Radio, Leana!"

She pivoted, snagging the two-way from Mkhwanazi's outstretched hand, and bolted out with Jit. Leana's steel-toed safety shoes thudded against the deck, their rugged soles gripping the slick surface as she surged forward, the radio's edge digging into her palm.

Day one, she thought, and a Code Blue's already clawing. Fifteen years drilled it home—crises ignored clocks. She spotted an old man sprawled on the carpet by the front elevator, alive but limp. Martha Franklin, his wife stumbled in behind, shrieking—her husband dizzy, then down, help sought from a nearby cabin.

Jit dropped to check vitals, her hands swift, as Leana faced Martha, voice firm. "Can you tell me about his medical history—now."

"Jake Franklin, 65," Martha choked out, tears streaking. "High blood pressure, prostate surgery booked post-cruise. He's got a catheter!"

Each word sharpened Leana's focus—time was bleeding out fast. The air thickened, taut as wire. Leana clipped the pulse oximeter on, prepped the glucometer, while Jit cuffed Jake's arm for pressure.

She muttered under her breath, "Airway clear, no pain, breathing steady, circulation holding."

Then Jake slumped, eyes blank, pupils blown wide. Jit recoiled as Leana lunged, slapping his shoulders. "Jake! Up, now—come on!" Her voice quaked, desperation clawing up her throat, heart slamming at the void staring back.

Lord don't take him—not yet, she pleaded silently, chest aching with a prayer she could not voice, every fibre straining for a spark.

Leana pressed for a pulse—weak, a dead line. "Still breathing," she rasped, voice shaking, "chest moving, oxygen saturation normal, but pupils fixed, dilated."

She locked eyes with Jit, firm. "Code Blue—now!"

Martha's wails pierced the air as Leana fought for Jake's thread. "Please—someone, anything!" she begged, raw.

Bystanders milled, frozen—help or hide? Ioana, assistant guest services manager, stepped off the elevator, cool as steel. "Ma'am, the medical team's got this. Come with me—let them work."

Leana jammed the radio button, voice cutting static. "Code Blue, Deck 6 forward elevator lobby—repeat, Code Blue, Deck 6 forward elevator lobby!"

Ioana braced Martha by the elevator, phone pressed to her ear and called her guest services manager. "Rosanna, Code Blue team, Deck 6 forward elevator lobby—now! Again—Code Blue, Deck 6 forward!" She flashed Leana a shaky thumb-up—call live.

Seconds later, the intercom roared. "Code Blue team, Deck 6 forward elevator lobby! Code Blue team, Deck 6 forward elevator lobby!"

Jake twitched awake soon after, eyes foggy, lost. Leana dropped to his side, voice level over the adrenaline pounding her skull.

"Medical centre, Mr. Franklin—we're moving you." His lids flickered, a faint nod all he could muster.

Dr. Gutierrez barrelled in, pulling Jit's focus from Jake.

"Doctor," Leana said, sharp, "pupils fixed, dilated, breathing intact—no pulse, then he snapped back!"

"Blood pressure?" Dr. Gutierrez shot back.

Leana's gaze hit Jit. "You get it?"

Jit blinked, flustered. "Uh, no—he was out."

Leana snatched the cuff, slapped it on, eyes on the screen. "Low—80/50 mmHg. Heart rate's 116, climbing. Hold up—Martha said catheter, prostate surgery after this cruise!"

Leana and Dr. Gutierrez tore at Jake's belt, jeans splitting to show a diaper—dark red seeping through, catheter choked, urine bag, a bloody pool. Panic surged, a shared yell ripping out, "Hypovolemic shock!"

"Leana, he's off the ship—now!" Dr. Gutierrez barked. "We're prepping to sail—I'm on with the captain. Captain Alejandro, Dr. Gutierrez here," he said, calm but urgent. "Medical emergency—needs disembarkation, stat."

"Copy, Doctor. Gangway's closing in twenty—can we push it?" the captain fired back, crisp.

"We'll hustle, Captain."

Dr. Gutierrez faced Martha, jaw set. "Your husband's health can't wait—hospital's the call, not the cruise. He's awake, but two days at sea could turn ugly."

Martha's nod came fast, worry carving her face. "Hospital—quick as we can."

"Appreciate it," Dr. Gutierrez said, voice warm but firm. "Grab everything—passports, insurance, bags. We'll get you sorted for disembark."

Martha thrust passports and an insurance card at Ioana, hands trembling.

Dr. Gutierrez swung to Ioana. "Get Customs and Border on this—send a crew for their bags, cabin to medical centre, now."

"Ambulance too?" Ioana asked, poised.

"ACLS ambulance, yes—go."

Ioana gripped Martha's arm. "We've got you covered—everything's set before you leave."

The team stormed into the lobby—suction, defibrillator, oxygen in tow—Leana's heart slamming her ribs. Dr. Srinivas stepped up as Dr. Gutierrez briefed Ioana.

"Catheter's bleeding out," Leana said, voice quivering, "BP 80/50, heart rate spiking at 116."

"Intravenous fluids—now!" Dr. Srinivas snapped. "Medical centre, stat—Rodrigo, line in; Mkhwanazi, Ringers lactate, one litre!"

Rodrigo's hands flew steady. "Line's in!" he called, easing the room's edge.

Mkhwanazi followed fast. "Ringer's hooked—running!" she shouted.

Rajesh, chief security, loomed up, stern but warm. "Stairs only—stretcher won't fit guest elevators."

"Right, Chief," Leana said, chin up. "Fast as we can."

Rajesh barked at his beefy security crew, "Clear the path—stretcher's coming through!" They shoved crew and guests aside, no nonsense.

Mkhwanazi and Rodrigo synced with the stretcher team, sliding Jake onto a sheet, then heaving him up. Leana's chest swelled at their slick moves.

Her gaze flicked to Jit, narrowing—Twelve years, and you still freeze? she thought, sharp.

"One, two, three—lift!" Mkhwanazi belted.

The team hoisted Jake, Rodrigo raising the INTRAVENOUS bag high, and they barrelled down six flights to the medical centre.

Ioana charged into the medical centre, hunting Roberta. "Passports, insurance—copies, now!"

Roberta churned out three sets, stuffing envelopes—hospital, ambulance, guest—fast.

Leana and Jit beat Jake downstairs, hitting the centre. Leana fired up the ECG, wiring electrodes, her heart battering her ribs with the clock ticking. "Jit, notes—go," she ordered.

Dr. Gutierrez strode in, Jake's stretcher rolling behind. "Leana, referral letter's on me—Dr. Srinivas, you're up."

Jake landed in the ICU room, stretcher thudding down. Dr. Srinivas spun to Mkhwanazi. "Blood—CBC, urea, electrolytes. I'll grab an arterial gas. Leana, ECG, now."

Leana wired Jake fast, breath held for the printout. She ripped it free, calling, "ECG's up, Doctor."

"Flattened T waves, U waves—low potassium," Dr. Srinivas said, "second IV-line, potassium 10m/eq over an hour—run it till the ambulance arrives."

Rosanna burst in—customs, border, port agent, paramedics trailing. "Ambulance is docked," she snapped.

Leana's jaw dropped—Rosanna's crew had wrangled ambulance and officials onboard in a blink.

Customs and Border stalled Mkhwanazi's blood draw, clearance pending for Jake and Martha's exit. The port agent bolted, snagging Martha's gear for a fast out.

"Roberta, referral letter—print it," Dr. Gutierrez ordered. She glared at the printer, silently raging under the crunch, the room holding its breath for the pages.

"Roberta, why the holdup?" Dr. Gutierrez pressed, voice rising.

Roberta's stare locked on Gutierrez, fierce. "It's the referral docs—this printer's choking!" she bit back.

"Move it—ship's departure's on you!" Dr. Gutierrez's shout bounced off steel. "Roberta, now!"

Roberta's hands stalled over the keys. "Jammed," she spat, her cool fracturing sharply.

Dr. Gutierrez knew a late sail would snarl the docks— traffic a mad tangle, every delay a costly ripple. The company's wallet hung in the balance, operations teetering on a razor's edge.
Tears brimmed in Roberta's eyes as Rodrigo slid in, tweaking the printer tray smooth.

"Fixed," he said, calm as stone, handing Martha her medical packet—three copies fresh. "Ma'am, this is yours—insurance, records. Ambulance and hospital have theirs; keep this."

"Thank you, son," Martha said, voice thick with frayed thanks. "God bless you all for saving him."

Rodrigo darted to Dr. Srinivas, passing two copies. Dr. Srinivas briefed the paramedics, clipped and clear.

"Male, 65, hypovolemia—catheter bleed," Dr. Srinivas said. "No bloods yet—Ringer's bolus in, potassium prepped, ECG flags hypokalaemia. BP's 100/60, heart rate 112. Hypertension history, prostate surgery lined up post-cruise, per his wife."

The paramedic nodded, grabbing the records, then they eased Jake onto the gurney, rolling him out fast. Jake and Martha disembarked, hearts sinking cruise cut short.

After the crisis, the team remained in the medical centre, the atmosphere heavy with silence, exhaustion evident in every face. Leana looked around, marvelling at how quickly this group of strangers had become a cohesive unit, saving a life together just twenty minutes ago, each playing their part—some better than others. Roberta had struggled under pressure, Jit initially froze but later diligently took notes, while Rodrigo, Mkhwanazi, Dr Srinivas, and Dr Gutierrez performed admirably, though Dr Gutierrez needed to remember to avoid public reprimands to maintain morale in high-stress situations, Leana thought.

Observing her team members—Rodrigo leaning against the wall, catching his breath, Mkhwanazi massaging her temples to relieve tension, Jit furiously writing, perhaps documenting events to process what went wrong and right—she raised both her hands behind her head, stretched, and said, 'We've been through fire together now, bonded by the experience of overcoming a Code Blue, even with a faulty printer, what are your thoughts, everyone?'

But inwardly, she wondered if this bond was fragile, if the next challenge would hold them together. Was

Gutierrez's leadership strong enough to guide them through inevitable future crises?

"Hell of a start," Rodrigo grinned, tired, but real.

"Too close," Mkhwanazi murmured, rubbing her neck.

Dr. Gutierrez blinked, then nodded. "Let's get some coffee, anything for this crew."

Chatter sparked as they ordered snacks, then dove back into cleanup.

Leana swept her gaze over the humming medical centre, lingering on each teammate—duty of a steady drumbeat. Disinfectant stung the air, blending with gear hum and far-off voices. Responsibility anchored her as Mkhwanazi neared, folder in hand, her South African lilt singing through.

"Leana," she said, "here's your handover file—everything for running this place smooth."

"Thanks," Leana said, easing the folder from Mkhwanazi, cracking it open—protocols, inventories, schedules spilling out. Her gaze raked the pages, soaking in the gears she'd turn to keep this place alive.

"Defibrillator—check. Crash cart, stocked—check," she murmured, ticking off her list. She squinted at a crooked bedrail, jammed up. "Fix this," she scribbled in the file.

"Looks solid," she told Dr. Gutierrez, inspection done. "Anything else before we sail?"

"Nothing jumps out," Dr. Gutierrez said, eyes locking hers. "I trust you, Leana—you'll run this tight."

"Appreciate it, Dr. Gutierrez," she replied, grin warm. "I'll keep our patients top-tier, no question."

Strength pulsed through her as she eyed the medical centre, ready to tackle the Majestic Voyager's unknowns with her crew.

Snacks hit—coffee shop haul—and Leana's pulse jumped at her chocolate milkshake's chill glory.

"Solid," Dr. Gutierrez said, snagging his cappuccino. "Meeting time—everyone's here." The crew dropped into waiting-room chairs, eyes on him. He gripped coffee and pen, facing them.

"Team," he started, chin up, "seven days ahead, and today we meshed—damn good. Rodrigo's out post-voyage, Sham Singh from South Africa steps in. I'm gone in three weeks—Dr. Osiris Rodriguez from Colombia takes over." He sucked in a breath, rolling on.

"US public health's sniffing around soon—port check. Gastro cases dropped; crew nailed response, under sixty minutes. Shoreside's pushing extra measles shots— outbreaks elsewhere. They'll board, dig into health records, med expiration, equipment lists—make sure we're clean."

"Last inspection?" Dr. Srinivas cut in.

"January this year," Leana said. "Lost a point—popcorn kernel in the microwave."

Jit jumped in. "Before you pick on me, it was my mess. Let me tell you, I made popcorn because the microwave in the mess was not working. They found one kernel, and all hell broke loose. They removed all microwaves fleetwide."

"That was you? Now I must walk all the way to the mess because of you," Rodrigo said jokingly.

"One final matter, Roberta," Gutierrez said, his voice low. "I regret raising my voice at you. Past incidents—ship delays due to medical issues—have weighed on me, as I'm accountable for our team. In the heat of the moment, I sometimes speak words I don't intend."

Roberta's face shifted from sorrow to a smile, as if she had been awaiting such words, and she nodded, suggesting she accepted his sentiment.

Questions?" Dr. Gutierrez prodded.

"Good afternoon, all!" the cruise director blared over the intercom. "Sailing's on—Lido Deck 10, midship pool party. Photo team's set for Statue of Liberty shots."

Leana's grin broke wide—Statue of Liberty calling.

"Nothing else? Meeting's done," Dr. Gutierrez said, firm.

Leana bolted to Deck 4, crew-only turf, catching the Majestic Voyager pulling from Manhattan Cruise Terminal—five berths swallowing giants.

"Beautiful, right?" Dr. Gutierrez drawled beside her, propped on the railing, cigarette glowing—Deck 4 doubled as the crew smoke zone.

"Yeah. Freedom, democracy, welcome," Leana said, seagulls snagging fish mid-dive, yanking her focus. Her fingers dug into the rail as his smoke twisted through the brine.

"I trust you," he said.

Trust—or a trap? "What's up?" she asked, voice flat.

"Shipboard Command's griping—Dr. Srinivas rocked scrubs on Elegant Night, no dress code," Gutierrez said, rubbing his temple.

"Team's saying he ghosts his phone, radio too. Claims he lost track of time after back-to-back shifts, but that's no excuse for sloppiness."

"HR document it? Corrective record?"

"No, it has not," he shot back, blunt. "Informal chat— him, captain, HR. Didn't escalate—his hands stay steady on patients. I smoothed it with the captain; he's quiet now."

Leana's stare sharpened, shoulders squaring with purpose. "He's learned, as long as patient care holds," she said, firm, locking eyes with Dr. Gutierrez. "I'm crashing—jetlag's a beast. See you tomorrow."

Nearing Deck 0's crew quarters, her boots rang steady, resolve burning. A crewmate tipped a tired nod—she returned it, sharp. Dr. Gutierrez's faith was a lifeline—she'd back him against Shipboard or Shoreside heat. Defending Dr. Srinivas, no formal slap, screamed his crew mattered.

The Majestic Voyager powered ahead, shores fading, unknown waters calling bold and fierce.

.

Chapter Two: First Sea Day

Leana twisted the key in the medical centre lock at 8:55 am, shoulders stiff from a night of rough waves rattling the Majestic Voyager.

The air conditioners' icy breath hit her face, causing her nose to tingle as the lights came on, revealing the dreadful sight: a line of crew and passengers, their faces pale and drawn, their bodies shivering violently with the ship's sickening roll down the long, echoing corridor of Deck 0; the air thick with a palpable sense of fear.

"Morning all," she said, voice steady, warm but sharp-edged. "Seasickness hit hard—I get it. We'll sort you fast."

Her gaze sliced through the crowd, catching a crewman doubled over, pale as death, heaving dry. She lunged, sick bag thrust out, catching his spew just as it hit.

"Follow me," she ordered, grip firm on his arm, steering him to an exam room. "You're up first."

She parked him on the table to be attended by Nurse Mkhwanazi, then strode back to the waiting area, safety shoes clipping steel. Rodrigo leaned toward a woman—Linda Donovan, thirties, first-timer—her husband, Chris, hovering close. Linda's eyes glowed red, cheeks hot, exhaustion dragging through her frame.

"Mrs. Donovan," Rodrigo said, voice smooth, "you've had nausea and fatigue since day one, right? Tried meclizine for seasickness, but it's not helping?"

Linda nodded, her throat tightening as she spoke. "Yeah, the nausea won't shift—I'm really losing it here."

"Anxiety can make it worse, you know," Rodrigo said, his voice steady and reassuring. "I think you should see the doctor. There's a fee for the consultation, and if you need medication, that's extra—not to mention any tests or if they decide to keep you in. Are you alright with that?"

Chris's hand settled on her shoulder, steady. Linda's gaze darted—husband to nurse—before she jerked a nod, scribbling her name on the consent form. "Okay," she rasped, pen shaking.

Rodrigo took her to the respiratory ward, rolled up Linda's sleeve and secured the blood pressure cuff tightly around her arm, the Velcro snapping into place. He pressed the stethoscope to her elbow with quick, confident movements. "Vitals are stable," he muttered, deflating the cuff.

Leana watched Linda grip Chris's hand, knuckles blanching, her breaths shallow as they waited for Dr. Srinivas. Linda's jaw locked tight, eyes glassy with fear, silent but screaming inside. Leana's gut twisted—she'd seen that look too often, passengers unravelled by the ship's sway and their own secrets. Linda's thin voice, whispered to Chris, "Sorry love, I will submit to my health insurance when I get home". Leana had a duty save lives first, but the bill loomed—a bloody axe over guests who just want to enjoy their vacation. Could Leana heap debt on despair, or pause. Not if it's life threatening.

Leana watched Linda grip Chris's hand, knuckles blanching, her breaths shallow as they waited for Dr. Srinivas. Linda's jaw locked tight, eyes glassy with fear, silent but screaming inside. Leana's gut twisted—too many passengers unravelled by the ship's sway and their own secrets.

Rodrigo rapped on Dr. Srinivas's door, brows knitted, then paused, glancing at Mkhwanazi. She nudged him, voice sharp with Johannesburg grit. "Go on, tell him straight—she's very ill, no time for dawdling." Rodrigo flinched, his Filipino instinct to ease into urgency—a nod to hierarchy—jarred by her South African bluntness, a candour Leana knew well from her Cape Town's wards. She caught the flicker of tension—same team, different beats.

"Doc," Rodrigo said, voice steady now, pushing past the hiccup, "we've got a case: Linda Donovan. First-timer, vomiting since yesterday, before we even sailed." Leana followed them in, noting Srinivas's sharp gaze lift, sensing the urgency. She'd smooth those edges later—keep them synced, no matter their roots.

Dr. Srinivas leaned forward slightly, his eyes narrowing as Rodrigo continued. "She's dizzy and lightheaded, with a mild stomach ache after vomiting all morning following breakfast. Her bowel movements are regular, but she struggles with nausea during episodes of vomiting. There's no fever, no cough, and no sensitivity to light."

Leana stood with her arms crossed, leaning against the wall as Rodrigo provided more details. "She smokes tobacco, drinks very little alcohol, and consumes little coffee, though she enjoys acidic foods. Complains of having headaches lately and takes ibuprofen or paracetamol for them. She uses cannabis daily and finds relief in alternating hot and cold baths; there's also a rash on her left thigh."

"She's also had similar symptoms before—vomiting during labour," Rodrigo concluded, eyeing Dr. Srinivas. "Since she's new to sea travel, I suspect it might be seasickness."

Leana watched Dr. Srinivas tap his fingers on the desk, his gaze sharpening as he thought deeply. "Take me to her!" he said suddenly, grabbing his stethoscope and rising quickly.

Rodrigo led Dr Srinivas into the room, with Leana following behind. Dr. Srinivas noticed their anxious expressions—deep worry etched on their faces—and offered a brief, reassuring smile.

"I'm Dr. Srinivas," he said, extending his hand first to Linda and then to Chris, shaking each firmly but quickly. "You're dealing with some tough symptoms. We'll figure this out and get you feeling better."

Linda's voice trembled as she spoke, hesitating slightly. "Thanks, Doc. I—I hope it's not serious."

Leana noticed Dr. Srinivas flicking his pen against the chart as he reviewed it, seemingly searching for something—perhaps noting the mention of cannabis use or the rash on her thigh. As Linda began to speak, she suddenly lurched forward, clutching her stomach and vomiting into the sick bag.

Dr. Srinivas's eyes widened as he quickly assessed the situation.

"Rodrigo—administer ondansetron 4 mg intramuscularly,
immediately," he ordered sharply.

"On it," Rodrigo replied swiftly, preparing the needle and administering the injection into Linda's arm. She winced, sweat forming on her brow, her face pale and her lips pressed together tightly.

Leana spent an hour at the medical centre, triaging patients and observing Dr. Srinivas and Rodrigo monitor Linda in her ward. For a moment, Linda seemed to relax, but then she heaved again, her hands shaking as she held the sick bag. Just then, Dr. Gutierrez entered, raising an eyebrow questioningly at Dr. Srinivas.

From her spot near the ward door, Leana caught Dr. Gutierrez's low, sharp question: "Why didn't we start with promethazine? She's still vomiting—she needs something to settle her stomach."

Dr. Srinivas's jaw tightened, a flash of irritation crossing his face. "Promethazine would knock her out too much," he snapped back, his sharp tone cutting through the room as he flicked a dismissive glance at Gutierrez.

Leana understood his logic—Ondansetron was the safer bet first, targeting the vomiting without turning Linda into a drowsy heap, useless on a rocking ship. But Gutierrez had a point too; Linda's relentless heaving suggested they might need more than one trick up their sleeve. She shifted her weight, silently agreeing with Gutierrez's push for something stronger, when Dr. Srinivas's eyes darted to her.

"Right, Leana—prepare promethazine, 25 mg for intramuscular injection," he ordered briskly, his voice grudging but firm, as if conceding only because the Ondansetron hadn't fully done the job.

Dr. Gutierrez turned on his heel and left the room without a word, his head shaking in quiet dissent, leaving Leana to wonder if Srinivas's pride had delayed a better fix.

Leana paused, syringe in hand, readying the promethazine injection, when Linda's hoarse voice cut through the room.

"Doctor, I've left something out—I need to tell you." Leana saw Linda's frantic glance dart to Chris, her eyes wide with dread, her whisper barely audible: "I've got bad anxiety—no proper medication. I took gabapentin from a family member—they swore it'd help." Dr. Srinivas's hand shot up, halting Leana mid-motion.

"Hold off on that promethazine," he said firmly, his gaze locking onto Linda as she pressed on, her voice frail.

"I got to the terminal at 9:30 yesterday morning and started vomiting soon after. Breakfast wouldn't stay down. The gabapentin stopped it completely for a full day—until this morning's meal brought it all back."

Leana watched Dr. Srinivas's brow crease, his jaw tightening as he mulled over Linda's words. He leaned forward, clearly weighing the mess of her self-medication against her current state—her cruise holiday teetering on the edge of ruin.

Linda's fingers twisted the hem of her blouse, her eyes flicking nervously between Dr. Srinivas and Chris, whose steady hand rested on her shoulder. "Could I have gabapentin with promethazine?" she rasped, her voice thick with desperation.

Dr. Srinivas eased back, his pen tapping his chin as he studied her. "We don't usually prescribe gabapentin for anxiety here," he said slowly, choosing his words with care. "It's a prescription drug—starting it on board without your doctor's records is dodgy.

Legally, it's meant for home, under supervision, maybe with therapy too. You've already had ondansetron—let's see why that's not holding."

Leana's mind raced—why hadn't Linda mentioned the gabapentin earlier? The pieces clicked: Linda's shaking, the nausea, the panic—it screamed withdrawal, likely from both cannabis and gabapentin. Stopping them cold could easily spark this mess. She caught Dr. Srinivas's glance, a silent nod passing between them—classic withdrawal signs, no doubt about it.

"Besides," Dr. Srinivas added, his tone measured, "gabapentin takes weeks to settle anxiety properly. Your vitals are steady—no panic attack calling for benzodiazepines yet. This might be withdrawal kicking in, not just seasickness." He scribbled a note on her chart, documenting her admission.

Chris's grip tightened on her shoulder, but Linda slumped, exhaustion etching her frame. Leana saw the spark dim in her eyes, her longing for relief clashing with the reality sinking in.

Srinivas entered the exam room, chart in hand, his gaze sharp but tired. Leana stood by, logging vitals, her mind churning—care first, or let the cost choke her call?

"Mrs. Donovan," Srinivas said, voice measured, "your vomiting's likely tied to withdrawal—alcohol, perhaps, from the cruise's flow. Gabapentin, 300mg daily, can steady your nerves, ease the shakes driving this. It's not a quick fix for nausea—takes hours, maybe days—but it might calm you, make you feel better indirectly."

Linda nodded, pale, clutching Chris. "Anything, doctor—I just want it gone." She swallowed the first dose, water trembling in her hand. "Feels… better already," she murmured, eyes hopeful, a flicker Leana caught—placebo, or desperation talking?

"Just for the cruise?" she pressed, her voice tight with hope.

Srinivas's brow twitched, his glance meeting Leana's, cautious. "That's reassuring, but it's probably just your mind settling down, Mrs. Donovan—gabapentin won't stop the vomiting itself, but it might reduce the queasiness and the feeling of needing to vomit." He scribbled the script, handing it over,

Just for the cruise?" she pressed, her voice tight with hope.

"Yes, but it's temporary—strictly for withdrawal relief," he said firmly. "You'll need to sign a consent form for this, and see your doctor back home for a proper plan—therapy included."

"Fine, Doctor," Linda said, clutching Chris's hand like a lifeline. "Whatever keeps me going."

"Good," Dr. Srinivas replied, his tone softening but resolute.

"This is a stopgap—only for the cruise." He slid a consent form, explaining, "It's gabapentin, 300 mg daily, to ease withdrawal. Risks include drowsiness, dizziness—any trouble, you come back immediately."

Leana watched Dr. Srinivas finish the prescription, Linda's chest rising and falling fast as hope wrestled with dread in her fierce grip on Chris. He held the paper out, pausing. "This isn't a fix," he said sternly. "It's just to tide you over." Linda grabbed it quickly, her trembling hands betraying her urgency.

"The pharmacy will have your medication," he added. "If it doesn't work or you feel worse, return here straight away."

"Thank you, Doctor," Linda rasped, tears welling in her eyes, her voice shaky. "It means the world."

"Anytime," Dr. Srinivas replied, his tone softening. "You're my priority—get in touch if it's rough."

Leana followed their slow shuffle towards the pharmacy, Linda's fingers crumpling the prescription in her damp palm.

The small, bright room greeted them with the clean scent of sterile packaging. At the counter, a Nurse Mkhwanazi looked up with a gentle smile.

"Hello," she said warmly. "I'm Nurse Mkhwanazi. What can I do for you?"

Linda thrust the paper forward. "Dr. Srinivas prescribed this—gabapentin and ondansetron," she stammered.

"Of course," Mkhwanazi replied, taking it from her unsteady hand. "I'll sort it out quickly."

As Mkhwanazi reached for the shelves, Leana saw Linda glance at Chris—his hand steadying hers—before she swayed, nausea hitting hard, her jaw clenching.

Mkhwanazi returned with the medication and a crisp instruction sheet and advised dosage instructions. "Call us if it gets worse", she said.

"Thanks," Linda muttered, taking the bottle in her shaky grasp. The ship's sway mirrored her churning stomach—she drew a sharp breath, battling the discomfort.
Leana watched Linda hobble out, Chris supporting her—her face a mix of resolve and unease. She'd push through, perhaps, with this small aid in hand.

Leana stepped in as Dr. Gutierrez examined Ni Luh Suantari, a young Indonesian crew member perched on the edge of the exam table, fingers fidgeting in her lap. Dr. Gutierrez flipped through her chart with a keen gaze.

"Last period—5th June," he said, checking the dates. "Today's 26th July—no pain or nausea. Here to confirm a pregnancy?"

Ni Luh nodded eagerly, her face lighting up. "Yes, Doctor—a home test showed positive."

"Congratulations," Dr. Gutierrez replied, smiling broadly as he reached for his stethoscope. "Let's ensure everything's progressing well."

Leana stayed and conducted the urine dipstick pregnancy as Dr Gutierez conducted the exam with calm precision.

Ni Luh perched on the exam table, hands knotted, eyes dodging Leana's as she showed the test to Dr Guitterez.

"Test's positive," Gutierrez said, voice low, chart snapping shut. "Early days—risks, but you're fit. We'll track it."

Leana logged vitals—pulse 82, BP 122/78—catching Ni Luh's wince. "Toilet's a bother lately," she muttered.

. "Just quick trips." Leana's pen paused—odd, but not dire.

Leana said, "There's no evidence of infection or blood in your urine, but don't hesitate to call if it becomes problematic."

"Ni Luh," Dr. Guitterez said, his expression turning grave, "housekeeping's demanding—lifting, slippery floors, constant standing. It could strain you and the baby."
Her voice wavered but held firm. "I understand, Doctor." Leana noticed Ni Luh's hands instinctively shield her belly, memories of heavy laundry shifts flickering in her tense posture.

"Cleaning chemicals are a risk too," Dr. Gutierrez added gently. "It's too dangerous—pregnancy leave starts after this voyage."

Ni Luh swallowed hard, her hands cradling her stomach. Leana saw a flicker of dread cross her face, the prospect of leaving her job settling heavily.

"Thank you, Doctor," Ni Luh whispered, tears glistening. "I'll do what's best for my baby."

"You and the little one are the priority," Dr. Gutierrez said, resting a steady hand on her shoulder. "I'm informing HR you'll be on pregnancy leave. You'll need to sign some forms."

He turned to Leana. "Zika form for Ni Luh—now." Then to Ni Luh: "Sign this with HR—I'll certify the pregnancy."

"Travel costs covered by me, Doctor?" Ni Luh asked, her voice faint.

"No, the company's sorting it," he assured her.

Leana handed her the form—Ni Luh's fingers brushed it lightly before she shuffled out, her walk stiff with mixed emotions, resolve now driving her to protect her child.

Leana's shift dragged on—headaches and seasick complaints piling up since dawn—when suddenly—the captain's voice boomed over intercom cutting through hum machinery background noise: "Secure all heavy gear—we're facing rough seas until tomorrow night."

She sighed inwardly knowing what that meant—more patients stumbling in dizzy disoriented—some injured slipping wet decks others vomiting uncontrollably again already overwhelmed medical centre bracing itself yet another wave literal sense too now not just metaphorical anymore either way though must be prepared to handle whatever came next because wasn't that the job after all?

Leana leaned against the counter in the medical centre, her arms crossed, as Nurse Mkhwanazi glanced up from sorting supplies. "Ever think the captain spares a thought for what his sailing calls do to us?" Mkhwanazi asked, her tone sharp with exhaustion. "This rough weather—crew stumbling in half-dead, us scrambling to patch them up. Does he even care about the strain we're under, keeping everyone going while the ship tosses like this?"

Leana's jaw tightened, a flicker of her own doubts bubbling up—she'd wondered the same bloody thing more than once today. But she straightened, her voice firm as she met Mkhwanazi's gaze.

"Look, he's got to think of the whole ship, hasn't he? Getting us from A to B safely, that's his job—efficiently, no cock-ups. Bad weather's not his fault; it's the sea's doing. He can't stop to nursemaid every crew member's sniffle or slip. That's on us—our patch to keep them afloat, literally and all. He's not blind to it, just prioritising what keeps this tub moving. So, yeah, it lands on us to sort the mess, but I reckon he trusts us to handle it—quietly, no fuss." She shrugged, pushing off the counter, swallowing the grumble she'd kept to herself all shift.

She glanced at an email—a Nassau port agent pressing for hospital payment details. "Dr. Gutierrez," she called across the medical centre, "Shoreside Medical confirmed that guarantee yet?"

"Not yet," he replied briskly. "Dr. Srinivas deals with Shoreside Health referrals."

Leana dialled Dr. Srinivas, the line ringing six times before he answered sharply, Roberta's familiar laugh echoing in the background. "Dr. Srinivas," she said evenly, "sorry to interrupt—dental referrals to Shoreside Health sent?"

"This?" he snapped irritably. "Can't it wait? I've just left the clinic."

Her tone hardened slightly. "Appointments fill up fast—we need that payment letter today to avoid a mess. Not critical, but let's get it done." She hung up, jaw tight.

Leana exhaled sharply, drafting a reply to the port agent—team copied in: "Still awaiting Shoreside Health payment confirmation. Dental bookings for three crew can proceed now."

While drafting a hospital update, an email from Martha pinged in—Jake admitted, surgery booked, and she thanked the Majestic Voyager crew for their swift action. A quiet pride stirred in Leana's chest as she signed off, her shift at last complete.

Chapter Three: Second Sea Day

Leana's phone pierced the darkness of her cabin at 4:03 am, the Guest Services label stark on the illuminated screen. She seized it, her throat dry and coarse from sleep, the remnants of rest still clinging to her voice.

"Lead Nurse—Cabin 6274, emergency," Keisha's voice cut through the static, precise and urgent. "The husband is in severe pain. The on-call nurse—six rings, no response."

Leana's grip tightened around the phone—twelve years of service, and Jit had failed once more? She pulled on her scrubs with haste, her boots striking the crew corridor floor, the hum of fluorescent lights grating against her senses like an insistent drone. Her fist connected with Jit's door—three firm knocks, the frame trembling beneath her determined strikes.

Jit's door opened slowly—her hair dishevelled, eyes clouded with fatigue, a tempest simmering in her expression. "What is it now?" she demanded, her tone harsh.

"Cabin 6274—emergency," Leana replied, her voice calm and measured, her gaze shifting to the nightstand phone, its blank screen a silent rebuke. She refrained from stating that Guest Services had contacted Jit first—her unspoken pause carried the weight of that truth, cutting like a finely honed blade.

Jit's chin lifted sharply. "I didn't hear anything," she declared, reaching for her phone—its display dead.

Mkhwanazi's door creaked open behind Leana, her voice gentle, eyes still heavy with sleep. "It rang four times—I heard it distinctly."

Jit's nostrils flared, her breath sharp. "Allow me a few minutes to dress in my scrubs," she said curtly, closing the door with a decisive thud.

Leana's phone vibrated against her palm as she pressed it to her ear, her pulse quickening. Before she could utter a word, Guest Services spoke again, the voice urgent and strained through the line. "Stateroom 6274 is on the line for you, immediately."

"This is Jennifer Roberts—" The words spilled forth in breathless gasps. "My husband, Jason—he is in considerable pain!"

"I'm on my way, Mrs. Roberts." Leana's pen scratched the cabin number—6274—across her palm, ink marking flesh in the absence of paper, time too precious to waste when Jit's oversight had already delayed them. She grabbed the medical bag stationed outside Jit's door, its familiar weight settling in her grasp, then dashed down the corridor, her boots resounding like a call to action.

Upon reaching the cabin, Leana discovered Jason contorted in agony, perspiration streaming down his forehead, his hands grasping desperately at his abdomen.

"Stomach's killing me," Jason said, clutching his side, voice rough. "Sharp, like knives. I'm on methadone—

clean a year, swear it." His gaze held hers, defiant but shaky, a man fighting old shadows.

Leana nodded, gloving up, her torch scanning his taut abdomen—no swelling, but pain flared at her touch. Her gut twisted—methadone flagged withdrawal risks, but his claim of sobriety begged trust. Duty screamed care—tests, scans—but judging him could cloud her call, miss the truth. "We'll do bloods, check your gut," she said, voice steady. "Methadone's noted—could be spasms, infection, or worse. Hang in, Jason." She logged it, ethical weight settling—care him right, or risk breaking a man clawing for redemption?

"Let's transport you to the medical centre, Mr. Roberts. We'll resolve this," Leana assured him, her tone steady and reassuring as she assisted him to his feet. She reached for her phone to request a wheelchair, her fingers brushing the screen, when Jit wheeled one in, its wheels catching on the carpet with an abrupt jolt.
"I'll take charge of him," Jit declared sharply, her gaze piercing the medical bag clasped in Leana's hand with evident irritation.

Leana disregarded the curt remark, guiding Jason's wheelchair alongside Jit towards the medical centre, her focus unwavering despite the friction.

Jit manoeuvred him onto the bed with a thud, swiftly attaching wires to the vital signs monitor, then dialled Dr. Gutierrez. "The patient's here—he requires your attention," she stated, her words brief and clipped.

Dr. Gutierrez appeared in the doorway five minutes later, his curls tousled from sleep, his jaw stretching in a mid-yawn crack. "Good morning, Leana—difficulty?" he enquired, rubbing his eyes with his knuckles, weariness etched into his features.

Jit hastened back from the ward, interrupting Leana before she could respond. "Two nights, abdominal pain—severe," she blurted out hurriedly. "No fever, no diarrhoea. Bowel function normal today. He's on methadone, former heroin user—last dose three months prior."

Dr. Gutierrez's brows furrowed, his eyes shifting between them in quiet assessment. "Leana?"

"Patient care comes first—discussion can wait," she replied firmly, her voice resolute, prioritising the immediate need.

He nodded once, stepping towards Jason's bed, his expression hardening with determination. "Good morning, Jason," he said, his voice calm and unwavering. "We'll alleviate your discomfort and determine the cause."

Leana followed Dr. Gutierrez into the ward, her fingernail pressing into her palm, a silent mark of her frustration. Empty intravenous trays and urine cups—unlabelled, left unattended—cluttered the surfaces from Jit's previous shift, a disarray as flimsy as her excuses. The sight tightened Leana's jaw; she mentally noted it for the next staff meeting, resolve hardening within her to address the lapse.

Dr. Gutierrez lowered himself to Jason's level, his voice steady despite the patient's ragged, uneven gasps. "We'll conduct blood tests immediately, Jason—likely keeping you under observation," he said, his gloved hand resting firmly on Jason's damp forehead.

"Are you comfortable with that?"

Leana's gaze cut sharply to Jit—her thumb scrolling through photographs of waterlogged chairs, her attention drifting elsewhere. Dr. Gutierrez, bent over Jason, remained oblivious to her distraction.

"Jit," he called back, his tone commanding, "establish a vascular line—immediately. Complete blood count, urea and electrolytes, liver function tests."

Silence followed—no movement.

Leana positioned herself directly in Jit's line of sight. "Concentrate," she whispered fiercely, her phone briefly displaying an image of a shattered lamp submerged in filth.

She registered Jit's retort— "My flat's flooded—a pipe burst, two thousand dollars lost, everything I own drenched"—her voice breaking with strain, her hands hesitating before seizing the tourniquet, guided by ingrained reflex. Her eyes wavered momentarily, as if envisioning ruined furniture and a life submerged beneath water.

Leana's stomach churned—she understood the toll such a disaster could take—but she gave a brisk nod towards

Jason, his fists hammering the bed, the relentless rhythm of his pain unbroken. "That situation won't remedy his condition," she stated, her voice low and resolute, urging Jit to regain her focus amidst her personal turmoil.

Jason's eyes protruded, wild with desperation, his fists clenched tightly, wrestling with the agony. "End this suffering!" he bellowed, his voice fracturing under the strain.

Jit inserted the needle, blood welling at the site, as Dr. Gutierrez stepped aside with Leana. "What were those hushed words about?" he enquired, his eyebrow raised in curiosity.

"She failed to respond to the on-call duty," Leana replied, her tone even. "Her flat flooded—a pipe burst. I suspect she's exhausted, not alert."

"That explains your presence—she faltered," he said, his eyes narrowing thoughtfully. "What's your plan? A delay in a Code Blue could have been fatal."

"Indeed, Doctor—she has twelve years' experience, no justification for this," Leana responded, her voice unwavering. "Counselling today, recorded in her evaluation. No reprimand—just documented our conversation."

"We don't need another Srinivas incident," Dr. Gutierrez murmured, his tone tinged with displeasure.

"Three weeks remain—the new doctor can manage him," he added, turning back towards Jason.

Leana observed Jit's hands—steady now, recovered from her earlier lapse—guiding the needle precisely into the vein. "Almost finished," Jit murmured, though Jason's features contorted further as she removed the tourniquet with a swift tug.

From the doorway, Leana noted Dr. Gutierrez pacing, his fingers tapping rhythmically against his thigh—could it be appendicitis, pancreatitis, or withdrawal? The blood results would reveal the truth, but Jason's constricted pupils in the dim light suggested detoxification to her, not sepsis.

"Enough," Dr. Gutierrez declared abruptly, silencing the monitor's persistent beep. He offered Jason a strained smile—his eyes stern, tension seeping through. "Twenty minutes—the results will come, and we'll address it then."

Jason's "Thank you, Doctor" emerged faintly, a hoarse whisper. Leana observed Jennifer's hand tighten around his—silent, her exhaustion evident from countless nights in emergency wards.

Jit brushed past Leana's shoulder, vials clasped in her hands, her gaze averted—her fingers trembling slightly as she labelled them. The flood's aftermath had subsided, Leana deduced, yet Jit remained burdened by its weight.

Jason's feeble groan pulled her attention back. Dr. Gutierrez adjusted the intravenous pump, his lips pressed into a stern line, paracetamol administered at a measured pace. "This will alleviate it somewhat," he stated, though Jason's restless movements conveyed to Leana that paracetamol offered scant relief against such intense suffering.

Jason's "Thank you, Dr. Gutierrez" grated through gritted teeth, his eyes reddened, shifting briefly to Jit—her hands moving mechanically, retrieving medications, avoiding eye contact.

Leana noted his fingers digging into the bed rails, knuckles starkly pale. The rawness of his pain stood in stark contrast to the monitor's steady tone—perspiration, tremors, a body locked in conflict. She had witnessed detoxification reduce men to such states before.

An hour later, the fluorescent lights cast pallid shadows across Jason's face. Leana traced a bead of sweat sliding down his temple, past a scar marked by old needle tracks, crudely healed.

"It still… hurts…" he croaked, his voice breaking, fragile as glass.

Dr. Gutierrez frowned at the laboratory results. "Normal," he said, his words heavy, unresolved. Leana detected his hesitation—his pen pausing, then swiftly issuing instructions.

The doctor's instructions were clear: INTRAVENOUS hyoscine butylbromide (20mg), INTRAVENOUS pantoprazole (40mg), and IM ketorolac.

Jit reached for the vials, her eyes lowered—her hands quivering, whether from weariness or remorse, Leana couldn't determine. Jason's sigh—grateful yet strained—filled the air as she mentally composed the incident report. His detoxification matched the standard profile—no narcotics permitted—yet his acute distress cut through protocol.

Jit prepared the medications, her hands gradually stabilising, while Dr. Gutierrez stationed himself beside Jason, his presence exuding calm assurance. Leana saw his jaw tense—he sought swift relief but was compelled to pursue the underlying cause.

"These should lessen the severity," he said, his voice low, confident, yet gentle. "We're with you—searching for the reason."

"Thank you, Doctor," Jason rasped, gratitude flickering through his pained expression, his eyes closing as the medications entered his bloodstream.

Dr. Gutierrez turned to Jit, his tone firming. "Monitor him until morning—no lapses."

Leana glanced at the wall clock—5:47 am, dawn filtering faintly through the portholes. She positioned herself between Jit and the cart, her voice quiet but incisive. "You're on duty until 9:00 am—consider it a reminder for failing to answer that call."

Jit's jaw stiffened, her eyes flaring with defiance. "The phone didn't ring—I was awake all night, dealing with the flat, insurers refusing assistance—" Her words spilled out, brittle and hurried, a woman worn thin, her twelve years at sea now overwhelmed by financial strain and water-damaged possessions. Leana's gaze remained steady; she pressed Jit's number—ringtone burst forth, echoing off the steel walls. Mkhwanazi had heard it distinctly at 4:00 am as well.

"The system records every attempt," Leana insisted, her thumb revealing the screen—red [4 MISSED] starkly visible and then phone battery dead–signal lost. "The signal was clear—no excuse of a poor connection and you keep your phone and radio charged."

Dr. Gutierrez stood prominently at the station, his coffee leaving a damp circle on the surface. "Leana—rest," he instructed, his gaze shifting briefly to Jason's motionless figure, then to Jit. "We'll address this matter after the afternoon clinic."

Leana discerned the strain in his tone—paperwork awaited, and her report would carry weight. She retrieved her jacket, feeling Jit's intense stare boring into her back, fierce and piercing.

Dr. Gutierrez exhaled heavily in the corridor, his breath laden with fatigue. "You could have handled that more discreetly."

Leana observed the waiters transporting breakfast trolleys towards the crew dining area. "Should we allow her to deceive patient's next time?" she retorted, her voice steady and pointed.

They parted ways towards their cabins. "See you in a few hours," Dr. Gutierrez murmured, his head shaking slowly, a gesture of mild reproach.

The clinic doors opened with a soft hiss at 9:00 am, Jit's expression dark and troubled. Leana noted the shadows darkening her eyes—five hours awake, three spent attending to Jason, unconscious since the ketorolac took effect. Jit thrust his chart into Rodrigo's hands, her movements swift and precise.

"He should have been discharged hours ago!" Jit exclaimed sharply, her voice reverberating off the steel walls.

Rodrigo—calm and composed—inclined his head gently.
"Take some rest," he advised. His tranquillity only fuelled her agitation; she stormed out, her scrubs rustling with evident frustration.

Leana turned towards Examination Room 2—Marian Thomas sat there, hunched, her fiancé's arm offering support. Red streaks radiated above her surgical bra, the signs of infection unmistakable across the bay. Her fingers twisted the gown tightly, her apprehension palpable.

Dr. Srinivas donned gloves with brisk efficiency. "The stitches have parted," he stated, his fingers probing the inflamed tissue. Marian flinched but held still—courage Leana acknowledged with a subtle nod.

"Blood tests first—then intravenous antibiotics for three days," he directed firmly.

"Blood analysis first," Srinivas clarified, "then intravenous antibiotics. A three-day course."

Marian's face fell, distress etching her features.

"Our holiday—"

"We'll manage it," Ben interrupted, his hand gripping hers firmly. Leana caught Dr. Srinivas's glance flicker—assessing them as keenly as he examined the wound.

The laboratory results arrived—Dr. Srinivas responded immediately. "White cell count is significantly elevated—metronidazole and vancomycin, administered eight hours apart." His pen scratched across the chart as Mkhwanazi prepared the intravenous line.

Leana's hand paused on the oxygen valve, her eyes fixed on the pump—1500 milligrams per hour of vancomycin displayed in bold red. Protocol was ingrained in her mind—600 milligrams per hour maximum—sufficient to alarm any seasoned practitioner.

"You'll feel better soon," Mkhwanazi reassured, securing the intravenous line with care. Marian's smile wavered as Leana approached, her own expression taut, concealing her concern.

"Switch to the new pump," Leana instructed, gesturing towards the device charging in the corner. "It's only a month old—let's use it."

Mkhwanazi's hands hesitated. "This one is functioning adequately—"

"Change it," Leana interjected, releasing the tubing clamp with a decisive snap.

Marian's gaze darted between them; Leana softened her tone. "The newer equipment is better and easier—best for your care." She adjusted the correct pump, ensuring the settings were precise.

Leana leaned closer to the station, her voice low yet resolute. "Fifteen hundred milligrams per hour—red man syndrome would manifest within ten minutes. Consult the pharmacology guide—" She handed it to Mkhwanazi— "six hundred milligrams per hour. Every instance."

Mkhwanazi's face flushed a deep red, mirroring the vial's warning label. "Dr. Srinivas instructed—"

"We identify errors," Leana interjected, her tone even and unyielding. "His included."

She seized the pharmacology leaflet and placed it firmly before Dr. Srinivas, its pages crisp under his gaze.

"You're correct," he conceded, his voice low and grudging. "It won't happen again."

"Indeed, it won't," Leana replied sharply. "Procedure requires completing the safety report. It was a near miss."

Dr. Srinivas retorted loudly, "You didn't administer it—it's resolved now!"

"No, Dr. Srinivas," she countered, her voice resolute. "I corrected it—you prescribed it incorrectly."

Leana stepped nearer, her tone softening yet retaining its firmness. "The safety report isn't a criticism—it's a team discussion to ensure we don't repeat the mistake."

Marian received the medication without complication—no adverse effects emerged. Leana monitored for any reaction to the vancomycin—none appeared.

Dr. Srinivas, noting her calm vigilance, said, "Return in eight hours," and authorised her discharge.

Marian's "Thank you, everyone" carried warmth as she departed.

Dr. Srinivas conducted the safety report alongside Leana, Mkhwanazi, and Dr. Gutierrez, reinforcing medical protocols until they were firmly embedded.

Dr. Gutierrez leaned forward, his presence commanding. "This ensures patients' survival—any questions, address them to me," he stated, his tone authoritative.

Muted voices drifted from Jason's room, drawing Leana's attention from her documentation. Through the slight opening of the door, Dr. Srinivas's whisper—"They're targeting me"—reached her, countered by Rodrigo's light evasion. The monitor's steady pulse couldn't mask their exchange.

"The lead nurse is excessively tense," Dr. Srinivas muttered, his back to the door. Leana's pen halted mid-sentence on her report. Rodrigo's hand rested briefly on his shoulder, his smile faint, his eyes lacking their usual spark.

"Forget the paperwork—the youth team's gathering this evening—"

"I'm meeting Roberta," Srinivas declared, his tone leaving no room for negotiation. Leana observed Rodrigo's shoulders droop as he turned towards the nurses' station, his customary liveliness noticeably diminished.

He met her gaze and offered a tentative smile before dialing Dr. Gutierrez. "Jason has been stable for hours—may we discharge him?"

Leana didn't require the other side of the conversation to anticipate Dr. Gutierrez's response. Rodrigo's pronounced sigh affirmed her expectation. "He insists we wake him for vital signs and nourishment."

"It's standard procedure," Leana remarked, resuming her report. The phrase Vancomycin error stood out starkly on the page.

"Patient care takes precedence over personal arrangements," she added, her voice calm yet definitive.

Rodrigo muttered under his breath, his displeasure evident, but he moved towards Jason, shaking his shoulder firmly—"Mr. Roberts!"—then forcing a rigid smile as Jason stirred with a groan.

Leana's pen struck her clipboard rhythmically—Srinivas's complaints, Rodrigo's haste, Jit's failure—issues to resolve later. Jason's drowsy blink drew her attention back to the present.

Jason's abrupt declaration pierced the medical bay's steady hum—"Oh, I need to pee!"—his voice still coarse from sleep. From the nurses' station, Leana observed Rodrigo respond promptly, his skilled hands detaching the intravenous line with seamless precision.

The bathroom door had scarcely closed before Jennifer stirred, rubbing her eyes awake, her anxious features easing as Jason returned, appearing more alert. When she proposed returning to their cabin for meals, Rodrigo's shoulders loosened slightly, a subtle shift Leana noted—the quiet relief of a nurse spared another hour of overseeing sustenance.

She overheard Rodrigo's conversation with Dr. Gutierrez, his tone measured and composed as he reported

Jason's condition. The doctor's approval arrived with the anticipated conditions—medication timetables, observation directives—all which Rodrigo echoed precisely while preparing Jason's discharge medications.

As Jason's wheelchair faded beyond the medical centre's doors, Jerry, a Romanian server, staggered in, clutching his swollen jaw, eyes gritty with pain. Deck 0's hum pulsed, antiseptic sharp as Leana set aside her charts.

"Nurse, I take painkillers a week, antibiotics four days," Jerry said, his Romanian accent thick, words clipped. "Doctor in crew bar says every night, 'Don't worry, dentist shoreside tomorrow.' Nobody calls—nothing." His hand trembled, tray-lifting agony plain.

Leana gloved up, torch catching a red, pulsing lump— abscess, infection raging. Her gut sank—no dentist aboard, just antibiotics stalling till port, and crew care meant company red tape, not swift fixes. "Jerry, you're on amoxicillin, right?" she asked, checking his file— Srinivas's note, vague, referral "pending." "I'll chase Shoreside Medical for that dentist—Nassau, tomorrow."

Jerry's eyes blazed. "Tomorrow? I carry trays in pain every day, nurse! Doctor says company covers, but I wait, I hurt—nobody cares. I go to Human Resource director if this is not fixed, I can't work with this pain." His voice cracked, a crewman's pride fraying, and Leana's chest tightened.

Duty screamed to ease him—find a clinic, push the referral—but Shoreside's silence and company penny-pinching could leave Jerry stranded, costs disputed if deemed "pre-existing." Neglect him, and crew trust would crack.

"I'm on it, Jerry—dentist by morning, antibiotics and pain meds till then," she said, voice steady, though doubt clawed. Crew deserved more than hollow promises, yet here she was, patching again.

Her screen blinked—no reply from Shoreside, referral stalled. Leana's jaw set, sensing Jerry's pain across the counter, a weight she carried. "Nassau, 8:00 am—I'll confirm it," she said, logging the call.

Jerry's nod was curt, his "Human Resource's next if this fails" a low growl, that crew glint hard in his eyes. The ethical knot twisted—care was her fight, but the company's chains bound it tight.

Her fingers were already dialling Dr. Srinivas when she glanced at the clock—1:05 pm. He was absent, likely at lunch. The call could wait until their meeting; Jerry's pain, though evident, didn't justify disrupting what promised to be another intense debate over documentation standards.

After an exhausting day, the medical centre's lights softened as the final guest left at 6:00 pm, leaving the sharp scent of antiseptic and a lingering air of unresolved tensions. Leana positioned herself at the forefront of the nurses' station, her fingers tapping lightly on the counter.

The team assembled—Dr. Gutierrez with his arms folded, Dr. Srinivas leaning against the wall with calculated nonchalance, and Mkhwanazi averting her gaze.

As Rodrigo made his way to the gathering, Srinivas leaned forward, his voice low. "Another late one, eh? You'd think after five years, you'd learn to pace yourself." Rodrigo stiffened but said nothing, the jab lingering like a stale scent.

As the meeting was just about to start, Marian returned to the clinic for her eight-hour antibiotic dose—the intravenous line administering smoothly, without difficulty. "Thank you, Leana and Mkhwanazi—reliable care," she said, her voice steady, placing her confidence in the Majestic Voyager crew. Leana shut the door for the three-hour infusion, then she and the patient quickly rejoined the team at the nurses' station.

Jit arrived and seated herself rigidly in her chair, her arms crossed tightly, her expression inscrutable.

Leana exhaled steadily, sliding the incident report across the desk with deliberate care. "Let us examine today's concerns—beginning with the unanswered emergency call at 4:00 a.m."

Jit's jaw stiffened noticeably. "I've already informed you—my phone didn't ring."

"It did," Leana countered, retrieving the IT logs on her tablet and presenting the record of missed calls. "Four attempts were made until your phone died. Mkhwanazi heard it clearly. The system registered it. There's no room for dispute."

Jit's nostrils widened briefly. "Very well. Perhaps I didn't wake. But that hardly justifies the manner in which you embarrassed me before a patient."

Dr. Gutierrez intervened, his voice quiet yet incisive. "This isn't a matter of pride. If a guest suffers a critical incident and no one responds, that constitutes negligence. Full stop."

Srinivas let out a dismissive huff. "And yet, here we all are, behaving as though Jit is the sole issue." His eyes darted towards Leana. "What of the vancomycin error? Or do we only record oversights when it suits us?"

The room fell into a profound silence, the air thick with unspoken tension.

Leana remained composed, unflinching. "The error was identified and documented. It wouldn't have occurred had someone verified the dosage rather than hastening the process."

"Hastening?" Srinivas straightened from the wall, his tone rising. "Perhaps if we weren't perpetually short-staffed, we'd have the luxury of your meticulous standards."

Rodrigo, ever the peacemaker, lifted his hands in a calming gesture. "Errors occur, yes. But the pressing concern is the lapses in infection control—uncleaned intravenous trays, urine samples left unattended—"

"So now it's my fault the cleaning staff neglect their duties?" Jit retorted sharply, her voice cutting through the room.

"No," Leana responded, her tone icy and precise. "It's your duty to adhere to protocol. Just as it's ours to prevent guests from developing sepsis because we failed to dispose of a specimen properly."

Dr. Gutierrez pressed the bridge of his nose wearily. "Enough. Starting tomorrow, we audit every shift thoroughly. No unanswered calls. No unhygienic stations. No unverified medication orders." His stern gaze settled on Srinivas. "And if I encounter another near miss due to someone overlooking the guidelines, Shoreside Medical will be notified."

A heavy silence descended.

Jit rose suddenly, her chair grating harshly against the floor. "Fine. But don't pretend the rest of you are faultless." She marched out to the operating room, closing with a resounding thud behind her.

Rodrigo let out a soft whistle. "Well, that might have proceeded more smoothly."

Leana released a slow breath, observing the strain that hung in the air like an ominous prognosis. "It's not about pointing fingers. It's about ensuring no one dies tomorrow."

The gravity of her statement rested heavily upon them. Beyond the porthole, the ocean darkened steadily—a silent testament that errors at sea offered no leniency.

Leana stepped away from the meeting's stifling atmosphere and caught sight of Jit in the operating room— her thumb pressing forcefully against her phone, her frown etched deeply into her features.

Marian Thomas's chart still required handover; her next dose was scheduled for 6:00 am, and Jit's shift extended until 10:00 pm. Leana placed the file firmly into Jit's grasp. "You're on duty until ten—ensure her stability."

Jit's eyes blazed, her teeth momentarily visible in a grimace. "Two hours overseeing an intravenous line? I've had enough of this," she snapped, her chair scraping the floor as she stood abruptly.

Chapter Four: Nassau

Leana pressed her palms against the clinic's porthole at precisely 8:00 am, as the Majestic Voyager secured its mooring in Nassau. The sun cast an orange-pink glow across the turquoise waves beyond, passengers jostling eagerly towards the gangway, their voices a muted murmur through the glass. She exhaled slowly—paradise unfurled before her, yet challenges loomed closer still.

Her thoughts drifted briefly to Cable Beach and Paradise Island—snorkelling, scuba diving, sailing, and boat excursions, all bathed in turquoise waters and pristine white sand. She had researched Nassau's history as well— the Queen's Staircase, Fort Fincastle, the Pirates Museum—grit embedded in her memory. The Straw Market pulsed with handmade crafts, festivals resonated with vibrant energy, and the locals infused the air with vitality. Nearby, Atlantis stood imposing—aquatic attractions, luxurious suites, lush greenery, and the constant hum of its casino.

Nassau drew crowds for its undeniable allure—beauty and spirit intertwined seamlessly.

Leana's lips curved faintly upward, her eyes following the disorderly scene on the pier. "A splendid day in paradise," she murmured under her breath, her attention catching on a cluster of people animatedly preparing for jet ski adventures, while a couple inspected vivid souvenirs spread across a vendor's table.

She turned to the referral letters, her fingernail catching on Jerry's—DECLINED stamped in bold red. Pre-existing condition. Her jaw clenched tightly. Dr. Srinivas had evaded her concerns a—now Jerry bore the burden.

"Leana!" Dr. Gutierrez's call sliced through the clinic's stillness, pulling her from her reverie. "Dental referrals—where do we stand?"

"Two approved, one rejected," she replied, a trace of frustration seeping into her voice. "Dr. Srinivas should have alerted Jerry—that his dental issue was deemed pre-existing."

"A harsh outcome," Dr. Gutierrez remarked, his brow furrowing deeply. "Nevertheless, we press forward. Has Jerry been informed?"

"Not yet—the email arrived moments ago. It frustrates me that Dr. Srinivas didn't clarify the coverage restrictions for him," she said, her tone edged with irritation.

"You care deeply for the crew, Leana," Dr. Gutierrez observed gently, his hand resting briefly on her shoulder in reassurance. "Now we must devise a solution Jerry can manage."

"Indeed," she sighed, her head dipping decisively. "I'll discuss it with him—find a practical resolution."

"Reliable as ever," Dr. Gutierrez said, his eyes softening with warmth. "We function as a team—Dr. Srinivas included, despite his oversights."

Leana marched off to deliver the unwelcome news to Jerry, her stomach tightening with sympathy for the young man. How would he react? What options remained? She straightened her posture, her commitment to the Majestic Voyager's crew fuelling her resolve—equitable or otherwise.

By 9:00 am, the medical centre crackled with strain, Deck 0's hum a faint pulse under radio buzz and chart rustles. Leana faced three crew members, her clipboard heavy.

"Morning—two of you have dental referrals, payment guaranteed," she said, handing envelopes to a pair of grinning stewards, who nodded and slipped out. Her eyes met Jerry's, his jaw tight, Romanian resolve hardening. "Jerry, Dr. Srinivas is next—hang on."

"Where's my referral?" Jerry snapped, voice low but edged, his waiter's hand clutching the counter.

Leana passed him the letter, her gut twisting as his fingers shook, snatching it. "It's been declined," she said, voice steady despite the sting. "Shoreside says 'pre-existing condition.' Dr Srinivas'll go over it, but—"

"Pre-existing?" Jerry cut in, Romanian accent sharp, eyes blazing. "I told doctor—pain for weeks, he says 'covered, tomorrow.' Now I pay? I'm straight to HR— Melissa will hear this!"

He stormed out, the centre's air thick, Leana's pulse spiking as she braced for the fallout.

Like clockwork, Melissa's call buzzed through, HR's tone clipped. Leana patched it to Srinivas's office, catching his sigh as he picked up. "Melissa, Jerry's referral was submitted, but Shoreside denied it—pre-existing, not covered," Srinivas said, voice flat.

"Srinivas, you promised him treatment," Melissa shot back. "Be upfront—don't dangle hope. You're new, but protocol's clear: check with senior doctor if unsure, not crew bar chats. He's paying out-of-pocket now?"

"Yes, I'm afraid so," Srinivas replied, a crack in his calm.

Minutes later, Melissa strode in, Jerry at her heels, his face flushed, apron creased. She faced Srinivas, eyes hard. "Crew health comes first, but they graft harder than you know—families waiting at home. Don't let them burn cash on your mistakes again."

Turning to Leana, she added, "He pays himself—final call. Next time, spell out policy limits, no false promises."

Leana nodded, guilt a blade—her trust in Srinivas's word had left Jerry dangling, crew care caught in company chains. "Understood, Melissa," she said, jaw set, the ethical knot tightening: fight for crew, or bow to rules that broke them?

Melissa called Jerry in, his anger a storm. "Shoreside denied your referral," she said, voice taut but kind. "You weren't warned, and that's on us, but it's declined—pre-existing."

Srinivas leaned forward, sympathy laced with strain. "Jerry, I pushed for coverage, but Shoreside ruled it out. Your Nassau appointment's set—dentist will give costs."

"Costs?" Jerry's hands flew up, voice cracking. "This is my teeth, not some choice! How much—hundreds? I send every dollar home!" His glare swept through Leana, Srinivas, the room—a crewman betrayed.

"We don't know yet," Srinivas said, calmly fraying.

"Your appointment is confirmed, once they assess, they will advise you." Leana's chest burned—, trust shattered. His complaint would hit HR, a mark on her watch.

As Jerry exited the office, his footsteps heavy with frustration, muttering under his breath, Nurse Mkhwanazi guided 82-year-old Robyn Mathers into the treatment room in a wheelchair, her husband at her side. The elderly woman pressed an ice pack to her swollen left knee, her face etched with evident discomfort. Mkhwanazi promptly recorded Robyn's history and relayed it to Dr. Gutierrez.

"Robyn tripped over a metal bar on deck 9 and fell forward, landing on her left knee. She was brought by the special needs team," Nurse Mkhwanazi explained, passing the chart to Dr. Gutierrez. "Special needs team reports she didn't strike her head or lose consciousness, and currently reports her pain as six out of ten. She noted a similar incident six months prior and underwent bilateral knee replacement surgery last year."

Leana caught Jerry's resentful glance from the corner of the examination room—his jaw tightening visibly as Robyn's wheelchair rolled past with a faint creak. The older woman's gaze briefly met the DECLINED stamp on his file, then shifted away, her attention subtly drawn to Leana's earlier exchange with him, overheard amidst the clinic's hum.

Mkhwanazi supported Robyn's elbow as she carefully shifted onto the examination bed. The heart monitor emitted a steady beep, contrasting sharply with Robyn's uneven breathing. Beyond the medical centre, laughter drifted faintly from the gangway, a distant echo of carefree enjoyment, while within these walls, the sole sound was the crisp rustle of paper as Dr. Gutierrez donned his gloves with a precise snap.

Dr. Gutierrez observed Robyn's strained expression closely.

"Very well, Robyn," he said, his warm brown eyes meeting hers with calm assurance. "I'd like you to stand and take a few steps so I may assess your mobility."

Robyn lifted her gaze sharply, pain evident in her tense features, yet she complied. With her husband's steady assistance, she rose and took five measured steps, her discomfort apparent but not incapacitating.

"Well done, Robyn. Now, please flex both knees for me."

She obliged, bending each knee smoothly despite the effort. Dr. Gutierrez approached, his hands gently examining her left knee. As he worked, Robyn glanced towards her husband, drawing comfort from his reassuring presence.

"My dear, it's painful, but I'll manage," she whispered, her voice quivering faintly.

"Naturally you will," her husband replied, offering her hand a tender squeeze.

"Very well, Robyn, I observe swelling on the front of your left knee," Dr. Gutierrez noted, his brow creasing with focus. "This is likely the source of your pain and discomfort. We'll endeavour to relieve it as best we can."

"Thank you, Doctor," Robyn replied, her voice hoarse with strain. Leana noticed her shoulders stiffen as Dr. Gutierrez continued his assessment.

Robyn let out a sharp hiss as Dr. Gutierrez pressed her knee, yet her piercing stare remained fixed on Leana. "That young man, Jerry—abandoned over a mere tooth?"

Leana's grip tightened on her clipboard, the edges biting into her palms. "Policy dictates the terms. A pre-existing condition excludes coverage." The statement felt cold and unyielding, like the steel instruments lining the clinic.

Robyn's fingers tore through the examination paper, the sound akin to fabric ripping under the strain. "Goodness.

One faulty joint, and I'd be in his position." The rustle of the sheet nearly muffled her words.

Dr. Gutierrez paused, his gloved hand suspended in mid-motion. "Is everything alright?"

Robyn's smile faltered briefly, unsteady as a faltering pulse. "Merely distracted," she said, though the falsehood was betrayed by her clenched fists gripping the torn paper.

"Robyn, I'd like to examine your lower limb for any loss of sensation," Dr. Gutierrez said, his tone blending gentleness with professional precision. "Please let me know if you notice any numbness or tingling as I touch various areas."

Leana stood near the examination bed, observing as Dr. Gutierrez carefully palpated Robyn's shin, calf, and foot. Robyn's eyes widened slightly, reflecting admiration for his expertise. Through the gloves, a soothing warmth seemed to emanate from his hands, even as they pressed against her swollen knee.

"Everything feels as it should," Robyn reported, a surge of relief softening the strain in her chest. "No numbness or tingling."

"That's promising," Dr. Gutierrez replied, nodding with evident satisfaction. He continued, "Next, I'll assess the movement in your ankle. Please point your toes downward, as though pressing an accelerator pedal."

Robyn followed his instructions, performing plantar flexion and dorsiflexion with steady effort, her movements unhindered. Dr. Gutierrez's expression conveyed approval, and he asked, "Does that cause you any discomfort?"

"Remarkably, no," she admitted, a tentative lightness lifting her mood.

"Very good," Dr. Gutierrez said, scribbling brief notes on her chart. "Let's proceed to stability tests for your knee. You'll feel me applying pressure from different directions, but I assure you, it will be gentle."

He conducted the Lachman's test, Posterior drawer, Valgus stress, and Varus stress with meticulous care. Leana watched Robyn's face, noting the anxiety that lingered beneath her appreciation for Dr. Gutierrez's attentive approach.

"Your knee appears stable," he concluded, his gaze meeting hers with calm reassurance. "I'd like to arrange X-rays to ensure there's no fracture or dislocation."

"Of course, Doctor," Robyn agreed, her heart beating heavily within her chest. "Whatever you consider necessary."

Nurse Mkhwanazi prepared the X-ray machine with quiet efficiency, directing Robyn's husband to the waiting area with a composed instruction.

The X-ray machine whirred to life, its low hum filling the room as Robyn held her breath, the images captured in swift succession. She tried to cling to the encouraging signs—normal sensation, stable knee—but a persistent fear weighed upon her, dense as a fog. Dr. Gutierrez reviewed the images on his computer screen, then approached her with measured steps to discuss the results.

"I have encouraging news," Dr. Gutierrez announced, his voice infused with brightness. "There's no fracture or dislocation. Your knee remains structurally intact, Robyn."

"Thank you, Doctor," she exhaled, tears of relief shimmering at the edges of her eyes. "I don't know how I'd have managed without your support."

"It's my responsibility to ensure your wellbeing," Dr. Gutierrez reassured her, his warm smile returning with sincerity. "Now, let's focus on reducing that swelling so you can enjoy the remainder of your holiday."

As Dr. Gutierrez presented Robyn with a prescription for ibuprofen, the clinical scent of the medical centre subtly faded, replaced by her growing sense of relief. The small white paper glowed faintly under the fluorescent lights, a concrete symbol of her fortunate escape from worse outcomes. Leana, stationed near the equipment, felt the disparity keenly—Robyn's relief stood in stark contrast to the burdens others, like Jerry, carried aboard this ship.

"Robyn," Dr. Gutierrez stated calmly and decisively, "I recommend you wear an elastic knee support and take a 400-milligram dose of ibuprofen every eight hours to control pain and inflammation." He gestured towards her swollen left knee, still pulsing faintly beneath her. "Additionally, apply a cold compress to your knee at regular intervals."

"Thank you, Doctor," Robyn replied, her fingers tightening around the prescription's edges, clutching it as though it anchored her newfound hope.

"Furthermore," he continued, "I would advise using a wheelchair for the time being to avoid placing undue strain on your knee," Dr. Gutierrez advised, his tone firm yet considerate. "This will aid its recovery and prevent further harm."

"Very well," Robyn agreed, her voice tinged with reluctance as visions of her holiday slipped away like grains of sand through her fingers. "If you believe that's best."

"Indeed," Dr. Gutierrez confirmed with quiet authority. "Now, do you have any questions or concerns regarding your diagnosis or treatment plan?"

Robyn paused, drawing a deep breath before voicing her worry. "How long might it take for my knee to heal? Will I be able to walk properly again before our holiday ends?"

Dr. Gutierrez regarded her question thoughtfully, his dark eyes reflecting a measured consideration. "Recovery varies between individuals, but given there's no structural damage, I'm optimistic you'll notice improvement within a few days. Ensure you adhere to the treatment plan and allow your body sufficient rest."

"Thank you, Doctor," Robyn murmured, a faint spark of hope kindling within her chest.

"You're welcome," he assured her, his warm smile conveying genuine care.

Her husband appeared in the doorway, his features etched with concern. His gaze sought hers, searching for confirmation of her wellbeing.

"Robyn," he whispered, his hand grasping hers with a gentle squeeze, "are you alright?"

"Yes, my love," she replied, returning the gesture with equal tenderness. "Dr. Gutierrez has cared for me splendidly."

With a soft exhalation of relief, her husband took hold of the wheelchair's handles and guided her out of the medical centre, the wheels rolling smoothly across the sterile floor.

The clinic ceased operations at 10:00 am, and most of the team departed to explore Nassau's vibrant offerings. Leana, Dr. Srinivas, and Mkhwanazi remained aboard as the designated port manning team—a compulsory rotation to ensure safety coverage while docked. The medical centre's abrupt silence felt jarring after the morning's intensity, the sterile air now interrupted only by the steady hum of refrigeration units preserving their pharmaceutical supplies.

Leana retreated to her cabin, securing three hours of rest before returning to reopen the clinic at 4:00 pm. The afternoon shift carried its own cadence—passengers trickling back from shore excursions with sunburns and twisted ankles, crew members slipping in during brief lulls between duties. She had just fastened a fresh pair of gloves when the clinic door flew open, silencing the air conditioning's low drone.

Jerry stood silhouetted in the doorway, framed by the blinding Bahamian sunlight, his heaving shoulders casting irregular shadows across the antiseptic floor. The tropical breeze swept in behind him, mingling salt and perspiration into the room. Leana's gloved fingers paused mid-motion, her eyes fixing on his flushed face and the tightly clenched fists at his sides.

"Jerry, what's happened?" she asked, rising from her chair and approaching him with measured caution.

"It's far too costly," he declared, his voice breaking with frustration. "I couldn't afford a root canal, so I had the tooth extracted!" He dragged a hand through his hair, the physical pain in his jaw mirrored by the distress in his eyes.

Leana felt a pang of sympathy for the young man, his shoulders slumped under the crushing weight of his financial troubles; she could almost feel the burden herself. She inhaled deeply, steadying herself as she resolved to investigate every feasible option on his behalf. "Let me discuss this with Dr. Srinivas. Perhaps there's a solution we can find."

She located Dr. Srinivas in his office, sifting through a disarray of paperwork. His brow was creased with focus, his fingers tapping restlessly against the desk, betraying an undercurrent of impatience or unease.

"Dr. Srinivas," Leana began tentatively, her voice measured, "Jerry's just returned from the dentist. He couldn't afford the root canal, so he had the tooth extracted instead. Is there any possibility we could request reimbursement for him?"

Dr. Srinivas paused, lifting his gaze from the chaotic pile of papers. He exhaled deeply, a weary edge to his breath, before responding. "Leana, I appreciate your concern, but it remains a pre-existing condition. The company won't authorise coverage for that expense." His fingers stilled briefly on the desk, betraying a flicker of discomfort beneath his composed exterior.

Leana's stomach tightened painfully, her thoughts swirling with the unfairness of it all. Why should Jerry pay for such rigid bureaucracy? She pressed her lips together, suppressing her frustration as she nodded reluctantly.

"Very well, thank you for your efforts," she said, her voice a hushed murmur, barely audible.

Returning to the waiting area, Leana found Jerry slumped in a chair, his face cradled in his hands. She sat beside him, her hand hovering momentarily before settling lightly on his arm.

"Jerry, I'm truly sorry," she said, her tone soft with empathy. "Dr. Srinivas confirmed the company won't cover it—it's deemed pre-existing."

His shoulders drooped further, defeat weighing heavily upon him. "I expected as much," he muttered through his fingers, his voice muffled. "Thank you for trying, Leana."

A dense silence enveloped them until the ship's horn blared overhead. The cruise director's voice crackled through the intercom: "All shore personnel, final call. Majestic Voyager departs in thirty minutes."

The announcement cut through the medical bay's sterile stillness, a stark reminder that the world beyond continued its relentless pace, indifferent to Jerry's broken hopes scattered across the clinic floor. Leana watched his shoulders sink lower with each word, his fingers carving fresh indentations into his palms.

As the clinic prepared to close for the evening, Jason Roberts was wheeled in, his face again contorted with pain. He slumped in the exam room bed, face ashen, clutching his stomach, sweat beading.

"It's worse," he rasped, voice tight. "Knives again— thought I was past this." His eyes, glazed, flickered with shame, methadone's shadow looming. With a thoughtful frown, Gutierrez told Jason they'd need a drug test and repeat bloodwork—a cautious tone in his voice to double-check everything.

Leana reviewed his chart; the blood work had returned, showing no elevated inflammatory markers or signs of infection. Although the methadone appeared beneficial, her instincts suggested his withdrawal symptoms were serious due to his past experiences. The results, given to Dr. Gutierrez by her, were then discussed with Jason.

"Jason, the drug test," he said, voice level, holding the printout: benzodiazepines, opioids, faint but there. "Positive, low levels. You said you were clean—talk to me."

Jason's jaw locked, then fell. "Before the cruise," he muttered, eyes down. "One slip—pills from a mate, thought it'd pass. Been sober since, swear it." His hands shook, a man caught, not defiant.

Leana wrestled with three choices: trust, support, or judgment—the latter risked his downfall. Duty demanded truth, but care meant hope, not shame.

"Your pain is likely because of spasms," Dr Guiterrez said, his tone measured yet firm. "Withdrawal has taken hold—methadone alone is insufficient if you've relapsed. We shall adjust your dosage and introduce clonidine to ease the symptoms."

Leana recorded the treatment plan, the ethical burden pressing heavily upon her—his relapse pierced her resolve, yet her decision could either save him or push him further into despair. The ship's medical resources were limited, with no rehabilitation facilities on board, leaving only her and Dr Guiterrez to mend fractured lives.

Dr Guiterrez continued, "Spasms explain it, Jason—your body's fighting old habits. Stay with us, we'll monitor." Leana handed Jason water, his "thanks" barely a whisper, trust fragile. Her mind snagged—care first, but his slip, her tests, cost him dignity. Was she mending, or judging?

Dr. Gutierrez's explanation ignited a furious blaze in Jennifer's chest, her face flushed crimson, tears streaming down her burning cheeks. She shrieked, her voice splintering with rage, "I poured everything into this holiday—every sleepless night, every penny—to celebrate your three months sober! And this is what I get? Lies? Betrayal? Do I mean nothing to you?" Her hands clawed toward him, trembling with a mix of heartbreak and wrath, her wedding band glinting like an accusation as she struck the air.

Jason's eyes darted desperately. "Please, just give me the same meds as last time—they worked," he begged, his voice small.

Jennifer whirled away, her wedding band smashing against the doorframe with a vicious clink. "Three months sober," she hissed, her voice a raw, venomous whisper, dripping with disbelief. She stormed out, disappearing beyond the threshold like a wounded animal.

Leana's heart thudded, her mind seething with the sting of Jason's betrayal—not just to Jennifer, but to the trust they'd all placed in him. The results flashed up: benzodiazepines and opioids, a toxic cocktail mocking Jennifer's devotion. Her own wedding band slipped from her shaking fingers, hitting the floor with a faint, bitter ping. She grabbed Jason's duffel bag and hurled it at him, sobriety pamphlets fluttering out—crisp, untouched, a silent testament to his deceit.

No one said another word. Jason was admitted, hooked to fluids and pain relief, his silence deafening. After four grueling hours, his pain eased, and he was discharged to his cabin—alone with the wreckage he'd made.

Chapter Five: White Sands Cay

Leana spotted Rodrigo leaning against the railing at 7:00 am, his silhouette framed by the sun's golden ascent. When she mentioned White Sands Cay, his usual composed professionalism faltered—his smile broke forth, sudden and radiant, like a beacon piercing the dawn.

"It's utterly breathtaking," he enthused, his voice brimming with delight. "The sand is soft and welcoming, and the ocean's hues—turquoise blending into sapphire— it's as though a painter crafted it."

As he spoke of swimming, snorkeling, kayaking, and horseback riding, Leana felt a phantom warmth graze her skin, the island's sun already teasing her senses. She envisioned herself tracing nature trails, binoculars in hand, spotting vibrant birds amid the foliage—a thrill she hadn't known in months stirred within her.

"That sounds extraordinary," she said, her eyes gleaming with anticipation. "Once I'm off duty, I'll certainly plan a visit there."

Rodrigo's smile widened at her eagerness, though he noticed her gaze flicker back to the navigation chart clutched in her hands. Her brows lifted in mild surprise, duty snapping her back to the present. "What about the first aid post on the island? My handover notes state that we should take our own medical supplies?"

He nodded, his focus shifting seamlessly to their shared obligations. "Indeed, we must pack our emergency medical kits—oxygen, suction equipment, an automated external defibrillator, and other vital supplies. We can't assume the island's resources will suffice."

Leana absorbed his words, her shoulders tensing as responsibility settled heavily upon her once more. Even amidst the island's allure, their duty to safeguard the guests and crew loomed paramount. Yet, beneath the weight, a spark of excitement flickered at the prospect of exploring White Sands Cay. Her fingers tightened around the chart, a silent resolve steadying her thoughts, could she balance both as this was her first time on this island?

"Thank you, Rodrigo," she said, her tone firm as she redirected her focus. "I'll ensure we're equipped for any eventuality."

The tender boat's engine thrummed steadily in the background as Leana set about assembling the supplies. Rodrigo's words lingered, underscoring the necessity of preparedness. She methodically packed the emergency provisions into a spacious duffel bag—oxygen tank, suction kit, defibrillator—each item a tangible anchor to her role. As she secured the zip, the bag's heft pressed against her, mirroring the burden of their purpose.

"Very well," she said, glancing up at Rodrigo, her voice steady despite the flutter in her chest. "That should cover everything."

Dr. Srinivas appeared at her side, his three gold stripes glinting in the morning light. "The boats are ready," he said, his voice sharp and clipped, cutting through the air like a scalpel. "Conduct a radio check first—particularly with inexperienced staff accompanying us."

Leana swallowed, a pang of uncertainty rising—his tone suggested displeasure at her inclusion, though his words held practical intent. Was it her inexperience he doubted, or something more? She straightened, meeting his gaze briefly, her pulse quickening.

"Of course, I'll see to it," she replied, her voice calm despite the sting. She glanced over her shoulder at the crew preparing for the journey, their movements brisk yet untested. "Thank you for the reminder."

Rodrigo's eyes glinted with a playful spark. "There's also a crew buffet area—don't miss the flame-grilled jerk chicken. I've heard it's exceptional." His broad smile widened as he envisioned the dish, the smoky scent of charred spices already teasing his senses. "Leana, I'll take your shift at midday, so you're free to explore the island this afternoon."

"Truly?" Leana felt a rush of gratitude entwined with eager anticipation, her pulse quickening at the prospect. "Thank you, Rodrigo. I'll be sure to savour that jerk chicken—and everything else the island offers."

"Excellent," he replied, giving her shoulder a hearty pat, his enthusiasm infectious. "Just ensure you're prepared for any eventuality."

As the tender boat eased away from the Majestic Voyager, Leana watched the gap widen, the ship's silhouette shrinking against the horizon. Her excitement pulsed vividly, yet a thread of duty tugged at her thoughts. Yes, she'd have the chance to roam White Sands Cay, to bask in its splendour—but her primary obligation remained the safety of the guests and crew relying on her team's expertise. Could she reconcile the two?

The tender boat carved through the crystalline water, leaving a frothy wake as it neared the island. A warm sea breeze brushed Leana's face, carrying the faint tang of salt. She glanced at her colleagues, each absorbed in their tasks: housekeeping staff stacking plush bath towels, beverage crew arranging bar provisions with precision, the technology team configuring the card payment system, and entertainment personnel tuning their instruments. Nearby, catering staff tended to trolleys laden with aromatic dishes, the scent of spices wafting faintly towards her.

"Leana!" Dr. Srinivas's voice cut through the boat's lively hum, sharp with insistence. "Did you conduct the radio check?"

"It's done," she replied, offering a brisk thumbs-up. She'd tested the communication equipment thoroughly before departure, its crackling confirmation still echoing in her ears.

As the tender boat grazed the sandy shore of White Sand Cay, Leana's breath caught at the sight before her. Azure waves lapped gently against the pristine beach, framed by lush greenery that seemed to pulse with life—a living tableau of serenity. For a fleeting moment, she let the beauty envelop her, her heart lifting—only to reel herself back, her fingers tightening around the duffel bag's strap.

"Welcome to White Sands Cay," said the island manager, extending a hand to shake hers. "I'm Victor, let me show you our communications setup, so you'll know how to reach us in a medical emergency."

As they walked, Leana's gaze darted to the surroundings—the swaying palms, the shimmering water beckoning her to dive in, the distant promise of that jerk chicken teasing her senses. Yet her steps remained purposeful, duty anchoring her.

"Here's our main communication hub," Victor explained, indicating a compact station equipped with radios and a telephone. "If you require support, don't hesitate to contact us. We're here to assist."

"Noted, Victor. I'll remember that," Leana said, mentally cataloguing the equipment's layout and protocols.

Leana exhaled slowly, her shoulders stiffening as responsibility pressed down anew, a familiar weight she couldn't shed. She turned to Dr. Srinivas, her resolve firm.

"Let's set everything up," she said, her voice steady despite the island's allure tugging at her. "We've guests to look after."

"I'm well aware of the procedure," he retorted, his tone clipped, irritation flashing in his eyes as he adjusted his stance, the gold stripes on his shoulders catching the light.

As they worked side by side, efficiently arranging their supplies and equipment, Leana couldn't dispel a persistent unease—a quiet whisper that the day might yet unravel. Whatever lay ahead, she steeled herself to confront it, her resolve forged by her commitment to her patients and a flicker of exhilaration for the uncertainties they might face.

The sun stretched long shadows across the immaculate white sand as Leana and Dr. Srinivas methodically organised the medical provisions in the island's makeshift first aid station. Palm leaves rustled overhead, their gentle cadence briefly luring Leana's thoughts from her task to the tranquil paradise encircling her—until Dr. Srinivas's voice jolted her back.

"Leana, the bandages, please," he said, his tone clipped yet focused.

"Of course," she replied, passing him the neatly coiled gauze, her fingers brushing the fabric. Her gaze shifted, catching on an approaching wheelchair. Sara Gough, a 78-year-old guest, sat hunched, her face etched with distress, her left ankle twisted at a jarring, unnatural angle.

"Dr. Srinivas, we've a patient," Leana called, gesturing towards the woman. They hurried to her side, sand shifting beneath their steps.

"What happened?" Dr. Srinivas asked, his voice softening as his skilled fingers probed the swollen area around her ankle.

"I… I stumbled on those steps while getting off the ship onto the tender boat," Sara faltered, each breath a measured wince. "It's terribly painful, could not bear any weight on it."

Dr. Srinivas met Leana's eyes, concern mirrored in his glance. "We must return her to the ship for an X-ray." He swiftly applied a SAM splint, securing it with precise, practised motions.

Leana watched, a quiet admiration stirring for his deftness, though her mind raced—how many more might need them today?

"Leana, will you accompany Sara to the tender?" he asked.

"Certainly," she agreed, seizing the radio. She contacted the ship's medical team with brisk efficiency, alerting them to the incoming patient, then turned to Sara. "Rest assured, we'll look after you."

"What a shame, I'm going to miss the stingray trip," Sara said to her husband, her eyes glistening with sympathy, "I need to get back to the ship."

"Will I recover?

Leana held her gaze, offering a reassuring smile. "We'll do everything possible on the ship to ease your pain and speed your recovery."

"Improvements are needed to ensure passenger safety while disembarking," she remarked while being escorted

The tender boat docked at the Majestic Voyager, and Leana handed Sara to Rodrigo, who lingered at the entrance, his expression alert. As the tender returned to the island, Leana stepped onto the shore, her boots sinking into the warm, powdery sand of White Sands Cay. She drew a deep breath, the salty air lifting her spirits as she braced for the day's remaining duties. Satisfaction warmed her—she'd ensured Sara's safe transfer—but now she had to rejoin Dr. Srinivas.

Approaching the small white structure nestled among swaying palms, Leana caught the sound of muffled laughter spilling from within. She pushed the door open to find Dr. Srinivas perched on a wooden stool, his arm draped casually around Amy Dawson, a striking dancer from the UK. Their shared amusement lit their faces, though it faded as they noticed her, Srinivas hastily withdrawing his arm, both sitting straighter to reclaim professionalism.

"Leana, welcome back," he said, his voice tinged with a forced steadiness.

"Thank you," she replied, suppressing a knowing smile as she glanced between them. "I trust all's been manageable in my absence?" Her thoughts drifted to

Roberta, Srinivas's partner aboard the ship. Should she mention this to her? A pang of doubt twisted within her—loyalty to her colleague warred with discretion.

"Entirely," Dr. Srinivas assured her, a trace of pride threading through his words. "Just minor injuries—nothing beyond our capability."

"That's reassuring," Leana said, relief easing her tension. "If you're agreeable, I'll take charge here. It's rare we get to enjoy such a splendid island."

"Are you certain?" he asked, gratitude brightening his eyes.
"Quite," she insisted, her smile unwavering. "Keep your radio close, though, in case I need you."

"Thank you, Leana," he said, his gaze conveying deep appreciation. "I'm in your debt."

Dr. Srinivas and Amy departed the first aid station hand in hand, their figures vanishing down a winding path towards the beach, laughter trailing faintly behind them. Leana watched, her chest tightening with a blend of empathy and unease. She understood the rarity of such fleeting respites aboard the relentless Majestic Voyager—yet a shadow of doubt lingered. Should she have encouraged this, knowing Roberta awaited him back on the ship?

Everyone deserves a moment's reprieve, she reasoned, settling into the makeshift office, the wooden stool creaking beneath her. If I can ease my colleagues' burdens, so be it. But the thought gnawed at her—loyalty to Srinivas clashed with fairness to Roberta, her friend and confidante.

The sun scorched overhead as Leana tended to the guests' ailments—smoothing cream onto sunburnt shoulders, wrapping gauze around coral-scraped skin. Her ears strained for the radio's crackle, poised to summon Srinivas if duty called. For now, she managed alone, the station's stillness amplifying her restless thoughts. Each bandage she applied felt like a stitch in her resolve, yet the quiet hum of the island buzzed with an unspoken threat.

A sudden "Ouch!" pierced the air. Leana turned sharply, spotting a couple approaching, their faces taut with discomfort. The man lifted his foot, a jagged cut weeping blood from the rocks.

"Excuse me, Nurse, have you any plasters?" the woman asked, her voice trembling as she sought reassurance in Leana's steady gaze.

"Certainly," Leana replied, her tone calm despite the tightening in her chest. She ushered them inside, deftly securing a plaster to the wound. "You might consider water shoes—available on the ship. They'd protect you on the rocks."

"Thank you," the man said, relief softening his features. "We'll look into that."

As they departed, Leana's eyes caught Jason Roberts and his wife at the excursion desk nearby. Jason's laughter rang clear as he booked horseback riding, his movements unburdened. Relief flickered through her—he was stable today—but the calm felt fragile, a thin veneer over lurking chaos.

The radio crackled sharply, slicing through Leana's fragile calm. "Dr. Srinivas, this is Roberta, do you read me?" came the voice, taut with strain. "I was considering joining you on the island—I will come with Rodrigo."

Leana's pulse spiked, her fingers hovering over the device as a wry smile flickered across her lips. She murmured under her breath, "Oh heavens, trouble's brewing in paradise." Her hand brushed her mouth, masking her amusement—and dread—at Roberta's timing.

Dr. Srinivas's voice broke through, hesitant and clipped. "No, Roberta, this sun is not good for your skin" The static swallowed his unease, but Leana caught the strain beneath his words. Her gaze lingered briefly on Jason and his wife at the excursion desk, their carefree laughter a distant echo, when a sudden uproar snapped her focus back to the first aid station.

A young man, Jamie Widdleston, stumbled towards her, cradling his newlywed wife, Celeste, in his arms. Panic carved deep lines into their faces. "Please, help her!" he cried, his voice quaking with desperation. "She stepped on a bee—she's having an allergic reaction!"

Leana surged into motion, her boots grinding into the sand as she assessed Celeste's laboured gasps and swollen features. She guided them inside, her heart pounding but her hands steady.

"What's her name?" she asked, forcing calm into her tone.

"Celeste," Jamie replied, his eyes darting frantically between Leana and his wife.

"Celeste, I'm Nurse Leana—I'm here to help," she said, kneeling beside her. The woman's throat constricted visibly, her wheezes sharp and ragged.

"Jamie, did you remove the sting?"

"Yes, but her EpiPen's in our cabin on the ship," he confessed, shame flushing his cheeks.

Leana didn't hesitate, seizing the radio while reaching for an EpiPen from their kit. "Dr. Srinivas, it's urgent—a guest with a severe allergic reaction at the station. Return immediately."

"Understood, Nurse Leana. I'm on my way," he replied, his voice cutting through the static, taut with alarm.

Leana turned to Celeste, plunging the EpiPen into her right thigh with precision. The woman's body jolted, a shudder rippling through her, but Leana held her gaze, searching for a spark of awareness. "You'll be alright, Celeste," she said, her voice a lifeline amid the chaos. Could she hold on?

Dr. Srinivas burst through the door moments later, sweat beading on his brow, concern etched into every line of his face. He dropped beside Celeste, swiftly threading an intravenous line.

"Leana, prepare methylprednisolone 125 milligrams and diphenhydramine 50 milligrams—intravenous administration."

"Yes, Doctor," she replied, her nod brisk. "Jamie, is Celeste allergic to any medications?"

"No, not that I'm aware," he stammered, wringing his hands.

"We must get her to the ship at once," Dr. Srinivas said, his tone firm yet gentle, though fear glinted in his eyes— mirroring Leana's own rising panic.

She snatched the radio, her voice sharp with urgency. "Victor, this is Nurse Leana. We've got a medical emergency requiring immediate transport back to the ship."

"Understood, Nurse Leana. Transport's on its way," Victor's calm response crackled back.

Leana's heart thundered as they awaited the tender, her mind racing through contingencies—oxygen levels, airway collapse—yet she anchored herself, her composure a shield. Celeste's oxygen saturation plummeted to 90% on the pulse oximeter, a shrill beep piercing the air. Leana's fingers moved like lightning—epinephrine drawn, tourniquet secured—working in seamless tandem with Dr. Srinivas's intravenous setup. No words passed between them; their rhythm was instinctual, honed by necessity, as the island's serenity mocked the crisis unfolding within.

Leana scanned the compact array of emergency equipment in the station, her mind racing through the steps for intubation should Celeste's airway fail. Her fingers twitched, itching to act.

"Housekeeping, Security," she barked into the radio, her voice taut, "I require assistance to transport a guest to the ship. We're short-staffed—only two medical personnel here."

Footsteps crunched outside, rapid and uneven, heralding the team's approach.

"Very well, Celeste," Dr. Srinivas said, his tone steady yet edged with urgency, "we're taking you back to the ship for further treatment. Hold on." His hands adjusted her oxygen mask with precision, though a faint tremor betrayed the strain beneath his calm.

The stretcher team—housekeeping and security staff—swept in, lifting Celeste with practised care and hastening her towards the tender dock. Her breathing had steadied slightly, oxygen saturation creeping upwards, yet the clock ticked mercilessly. Dr. Srinivas followed, securing the mask as they reached the boat.

"Housekeeping and Security are trained in resuscitation," Dr. Srinivas said, his voice firm as he dragged a sleeve across his sweat-dampened brow, the motion betraying a faint tremor.

The radio sputtered to life, Rodrigo's voice cutting through. "Rodrigo here, en route from the ship to relieve you."

"Her oxygen saturations reached 94%—you can escort her on the tender," Srinivas added, his shoulders loosening almost imperceptibly. A fleeting glint of relief softened his eyes as he cast a quick glance towards the horizon— Roberta's domain aboard the ship, a confrontation narrowly sidestepped. His breath steadied, the weight of her absence lifting subtly from his frame.

Leana's fingers tightened around the spare epinephrine injector in her pocket, its chilled surface anchoring her racing pulse. She edged closer, the acrid tang of antiseptic on his scrubs sharp in her nostrils. "Doctor," she murmured, her voice a hushed blade, "one physician, one critical patient, ten minutes across open water." Her thumb traced the dose indicator, a tacit admonition. "If she worsens mid-journey, it's your licence on the line."

His jaw tightened, a muscle pulsing as he accepted the emergency kit from her—extra epinephrine injectors, the defibrillator, a fresh oxygen cylinder. The foam bore the imprint of her grip, a testament to her resolve. "Ten minutes," she pressed, her gaze locking with his. "Not a moment longer."

A shout pierced the air from the dock. Rodrigo stood poised at the tender's rail, his medical kit unzipped and primed—Roberta beside him, her frame stiff against the ship's hull, a storm brewing in her stance. Leana's stomach twisted sharply, a cold dread seeping in. Had Roberta caught their earlier words? Without hesitation, she leaped aboard, the deck lurching beneath her boots as she gripped the handrail. Dr. Srinivas followed, his breath catching, then easing as his gaze settled on Roberta. Relief flickered across his taut features—confrontation delayed, and the ship's familiar order beckoned. His shoulders softened, a fleeting calm amidst the chaos.

"Change of plan," she declared, positioning herself at Celeste's head, her watch glinting as she checked the time. "I'm coming with you." Her shoulder brushed Dr. Srinivas's arm—a fleeting, professional touch laden with unspoken trust—as she reached for the pulse oximeter, its beep steadying her focus.

As the tender pulled away, Celeste's eyes fluttered open, a faint smile trembling on her lips in response to Leana's earlier reassurance. "You'll be alright, Celeste," Leana said, her voice a quiet anchor amid the engine's roar.

Jamie, clutching his wife's hand, fought back tears, his grip a lifeline on their honeymoon now shadowed by a crisis.

Leana watched White Sands Cay fade into the horizon, her heart hammering against her ribs. Every second was a gamble, yet she trusted Dr. Srinivas—and herself—to see this through. His relief had been palpable, a brief exhale as Roberta remained aboard, confrontation deferred. But

Leana's mind churned—would that respite hold, or would Roberta's fury await them still? For now, Celeste's shallow breaths demanded her all.

Dr. Gutierrez's gloved hands moved with meticulous care as he examined Sara Gough's swollen ankle, his fingers probing the tender flesh. A gurney clattered through the medical centre's entrance, escorted by two housekeeping stewards, Celeste Warriner's pallid face barely visible beneath the oxygen mask strapped across her mouth.

"Anaphylaxis incoming!" Leana's voice sliced through the tumult, sharp and unwavering.

Dr. Gutierrez tore off his gloves mid-motion, abandoning the ankle. "The ICU's prepared!" he barked as the team surged into action. Mkhwanazi was already wrenching open crash cart drawers, Leana's hands steady as she maintained pressure on Celeste's intravenous site, blood smearing faintly against her wrist.

Monitor leads coiled across the floor like serpents as Dr. Srinivas assumed control, his presence a quiet anchor amid the storm. "Oxygen saturation first, albuterol nebulisation! Leana, secure an 18-gauge line as well!"

His calm voice stood in stark relief against the monitors' shrill beeps and Celeste's jagged, gasping breaths, a composure honed by relief—Roberta's confrontation deferred, the ship's order restored beneath his feet.

Leana's hands danced in unison, the nebuliser mask adjusted, pulse oximeter clamped onto Celeste's finger. The numbers flickered upward: 93%… 94%… The albuterol nebulizer hissed into life, a fine mist curling around Celeste's face as her respiratory rate eased from 28 to 22 breaths per minute.

"You're doing brilliantly, Celeste," Leana murmured, brushing seawater from the woman's temples with a gauze pad, her touch gentle yet firm. The heart monitor's steady ping signalled a fragile triumph, though her pulse still thrummed with the weight of what might have been.

As Dr. Srinivas oversaw Celeste's stabilisation, Dr. Gutierrez withdrew, his gaze shifting to Sara. The medical centre's crisp air—20°C against the Bahamian oppressive heat—carried the mingled scents of antiseptic and unspoken strain, a stark contrast to the island's deceptive calm.

"Leana," he said, his voice hushed but insistent, "once you're finished, let Mkhwanazi take over here. Join me with the guest in the treatment room."

"Very well," she replied, her tone clipped. "Let me enter her notes into the system—I'll be there shortly."

The treatment room door sealed shut with a soft hiss as Leana stepped inside. Sara's medical chart landing on the stainless-steel trolley with a resounding thud.

"That stairway was a peril!" Sara's voice splintered the air, raw with indignation. Her knuckles blanched as she gripped the bed rails, her frail frame trembling. I shouldn't have to pay for this because of the ship's negligence; my lawyers will—

"Mrs. Gough," Leana interjected, stepping to the bed's foot where Sara could meet her eyes. "I'm Leana, we met at the island earlier. I deeply regret this marred, what should be a restful holiday." She eased Sara's injured leg onto a foam block, her fingers gauging the swelling's heat and breadth—could it be more than a sprain? "We'll ensure your comfort and a swift return to enjoying your cruise. We will have our security here to investigate the injury."

Dr. Gutierrez approached, his gloved hand poised above the misshapen ankle. "I see you have travel insurance, and it should cover you for this incident," he said, his voice low yet resolute, a penlight casting stark shadows across the bruising.

"Well again, I don't see why I should pay," she retorted

Leana intervened, "Mrs Gough–once we are done, our security team will investigate the incident and if they indicate that it was the ship's negligence, the medical charges would be waived."

He nodded to Leana, who was already aligning the portable X-ray machine, its hum filling the room. "We need three views: anteroposterior, lateral, and mortise."

The X-ray machine hummed into action, its low drone filling the cramped treatment room. Leana draped the lead apron over Sara's abdomen, her movements precise despite the tension coiling in her shoulders. "Please remain still… and hold." The shutter snapped, a crisp sound in the stillness. She shifted for the next angles, her jaw tightening as the narrow operating bed resisted her efforts—its confines a stubborn foe, thwarting her every adjustment. Could this day test her any further?

Dr. Gutierrez studied the digital images on the monitor. "Lateral malleolus fracture." He turned to Sara, his shoulders squaring. "We'll reduce and cast it now. You'll feel pressure, but the worst is over."

Leana prepped the plaster cast, cast padding , the chemical scent of activated resin sharp in the air. She caught Sara's flinch as Dr. Gutierrez manipulated the ankle back into alignment.

"Breathe through it," Leana coached, pressing an ice pack into Sara's free hand. "Squeeze this when it stings."

As Dr Gutierrez began to reposition her ankle, Sara clenched her teeth, bracing herself for the discomfort. She felt the pressure of his hands on her ankle, followed by an unsettling tug and a brief wave of pain. It was over before she could even let out a gasp.

"See?" Dr Gutierrez said, glancing up at her momentarily as he applied the cast. "Not so bad, right?"

Sara forced a smile, though her eyes betrayed her lingering anxiety. "I suppose," she muttered.

Leana watched the final layer of casting set around Sara's ankle, the chemical scent of curing resin sharp in her nostrils. As Dr. Gutierrez trimmed the excess casting material, she saw Sara's gaze flick toward the porthole where the tender boats docked—her jaw working like she was rehearsing arguments.

Still thinking about that gangway, Leana noted, snapping off her gloves. "We will give you some pain medication that will help with the swelling," she said.

Sara's fingers trembled against the cast, her thumbnail picking at the wrapping. "How long until I can—"

"You'll require follow-up with an orthopaedic specialist upon disembarkation," Dr. Gutierrez said, his pen still moving across the chart. "We'll conduct daily reassessments until then to monitor healing progress.

Leana caught the way Sara's shoulders stiffened at the word daily—the unspoken question about charges hanging between them. She adjusted the pillow under Sara's leg, her voice deliberately even. "Security will be in shortly to collect your statement. Let's focus on keeping you comfortable."

As she helped Sara sit up, Leana recognized that tight-lipped expression—the grudging acceptance of patients who knew the system moved slower than their anger. The cruise itinerary on the wall caught Sara's eye, her fingers twitching toward the highlighted excursion dates.

Leana noted Sara's gaze lingering on the excursion calendar—a small victory. She's looking beyond the injury, Leana observed as she gathered the discharge forms. The paperwork would have to wait; Chief Security Officer Rajesh Singh and his deputy entered with incident report tablets in hand. Leana stepped back, surrendering the space for their official inquiry about the gangway incident.

After recording the incident, Rajesh communicated with Leana and Dr. Guitterez, Rajesh confirmed Sara lost her balance on the wet stairs due to a combination of the tender's natural swaying and her wearing smooth-soled flip-flops, which provided inadequate traction. While environmental factors (wet surfaces and vessel movement) contributed, the primary cause was her inappropriate footwear. A full assessment confirmed that all standard safety measures—including non-slip stair surfaces, crew assistance protocols, and passenger advisories on proper attire—were properly followed. As such, the incident resulted from foreseeable personal risk rather than any negligence by the ship or its tender operators.

As Security stepped out, Dr. Gutierrez examined Sara's finished ankle cast with a practiced gaze. "You're cleared for limited mobility," he said, peeling off his gloves. "But you'll need daily check-ups in the medical centre."

"Thank you, Doctor," Sara murmured, forcing gratitude through the pain. "That security officer was very thorough—he even photographed my shoes." She gingerly shifted her weight onto the cast, wincing. "Now my trip is ruined," she added quietly, more to herself than to the doctor.

"Here are your crutches," said Dr Gutierrez with a kind smile as he handed them over. "You can use them to move around your stateroom, but please use the wheelchair if you leave your room."

"Feeling any better, Sara?" Leana asked, trying to bring some semblance of normalcy to the suddenly chaotic room.

"Um, yes, much better now," Sara replied, her voice shaky but grateful. She glanced at her ankle, surprised by its weightlessness. "I can't feel any pain anymore."

"Good," Dr Gutierrez said, smiling. He handed her a bottle of acetaminophen. "Take these as needed for any discomfort and remember to follow up with me daily." Leana assisted Sara onto the wheelchair and wheeled her to the nurses' station to sign the discharge documents.

"Thank you, Doctor," Sara said, her eyes darting back to Celeste, who was now visibly improving – her breathing steadier and her voice returning.

"Everything will be alright," Dr Gutierrez assured her, casting a reassuring glance at both Sara and the recovering Celeste. "Now, please, rest up and let us manage this."

Leana observed Sara's at the nurse's station as she watched Celeste in the ICU. The older woman's earlier scowl had softened into something more contemplative - fingers now absently tracing the edge of her cast rather than pounding it.

Back in the ICU, Celeste's oxygen levels returned to the normal range and her breathing had drastically improved. She was talking and smiling, which were both encouraging signs.

Jamie looked at the medical team and said, "Good job, Doctor. You saved her life."

Dr Srinivas smiled and nodded in response.

Celeste remained under close observation while the medical staff reminded her of the importance of always carrying an EpiPen with her.

Rodrigo's silhouette appeared in the medical centre doorway just as the ship's horn signalled the last tender arrival. He took in the scene - Celeste sitting upright, picking at a tray of bland hospital food but breathing easily.

Leana met him at the threshold, her gloved hand briefly squeezing his forearm. "Good timing," she murmured. "Your fast response on the island gave us the critical window we needed."

Celeste put down her food and hugged Leana, telling her it had been a terrifying experience and thanking her for saving her life.

"My dear, all that matters is that you are well now and able to enjoy your vacation," Leana replied.

Dr Srinivas then walked into the conversation, interrupting their exchange and asking if Leana had informed Celeste about any medical charges incurred because of the emergency.

"No, Dr Srinivas, I have discussed no fees because of the nature of the situation," she answered.

Jamie and Celeste glanced at one another; they were newlyweds without enough money to cover such costs.

Leana addressed Celeste and Jamie politely. "In the event of an emergency, the priority is to stabilise guests and medical bills are not discussed until then," she informed them.

"Once we've stabilised you, we'll explain the process going forward."

Jamie was astounded. "If I'm paying for a service, I should at least know what I'm paying for!" he exclaimed. Then he asked why a doctor wasn't immediately available and Leana explained that they had summoned the doctor by radio on the island.

Celeste enquired if they accepted personal health insurance and Leana replied no, but added that they provided receipts along with medical notes so guests could try to reclaim charges from their insurance companies.

The news crushed Celeste and Jamie's spirits. Jamie angrily chided Celeste for not carrying an EpiPen. Jamie admitted they lacked the funds to cover these costs and threatened to file a complaint about the lack of prior notification of medical charges.

Leana remained level-headed and consoled them, "It's only in your best interest that we act quickly in life-or-death situations. You always have the right to complain or dispute any charges before signing."

Are we done here? Can we leave?" Jamie declared.

Dr Srinivas walked in and stated, "yes we can discharge her, everything seems to be fine, breathing is normal, vitals stable, follow up if you require any further assistance and don't forget to carry that epi-pen."

"My apologies for not explaining the medical expenses to you first," Leana said as she took out the intravenous port.

"I apologise for my husband's attitude. I'll talk to him and don't worry–I'll pay the bill," Celeste replied.

Celeste's left the medical centre walking, a contrast to earlier; Leana watched her as Robyn Mathers arrived for her check-up, the memory of Deck 9's fall still a painful reminder, and Jerry's rejection echoing in her mind.

Robyn's wheelchair creaked, pushed by her husband, Harold, his eyes weary but steady, a quiet anchor.

Robyn, 82, sat tall, left knee snug in an elastic brace, swelling faded, her face less carved by pain. "Better, love," she said, voice frail yet fierce, shifting her ice pack. "Sore, though—can't stand proper. What's next?"

Leana scanned the notes—X-ray clear, ibuprofen 400mg holding, brace fitted yesterday for stability post-swelling, Srinivas's call to dodge a cast for now.

"You're mending, Robyn," Leana said, voice firm, though her gut knotted—care was working, but that bloody Deck 9 bar gnawed, a company cock-up buried.

"Swelling's near gone; brace until you return home, ibuprofen as needed, then orthopaedist at home. Wheelchair's safest till then." Duty burned—Robyn's legs deserved saving—but the fall's fault festered. The security report noted the hazard, yet pushing it meant legal fires, risking the team.

"Request assistance if needed, and retrieve your medical notes when you disembark," she instructed, burdened by ethical concerns—her comforting touch eased Robyn's pain, yet the firm's negligence persisted, a debt she couldn't repay.

Harold's nod was gentle, his "solicitor's on it" a low hum. Robyn's eyes locked on Leana's, sharp as steel despite her years.

"Shouldn't have been a bar," she murmured, voice cutting. Leana's breath caught—care delivered, but the company's lapse scorched, Robyn's grit a spark against it. She logged the visit, hope a stubborn ember in the ship's cold steel.

"My apologies, ma'am, the injury is documented by security, who can furnish you with a report," Leana stated, attempting to reduce the tension.

Chapter Six: Freeport

Leana stood at the medical centre's counter at 6:00 am, her coffee steaming untouched beneath Deck 0's muted fluorescent glow. The Majestic Voyager swayed gently against Freeport's pier, the Bahamas dawn seeping orange through the porthole—a fragile whisper of respite after four relentless days. She rolled her shoulders, the ache settling deep—fifteen years at sea, twelve as lead nurse, and the burden clung like a second skin, familiar yet unyielding. Her fingers brushed the mug's rim when the radio jolted to life.

"Cabin 8136, guest struggling to breathe," Rodrigo gasped, bursting through the doorway, his silhouette harsh against the corridor's glare. His scrubs hung damp with exertion, jaw clenched tight from a five-year stint capped by this breathless dash.

The mug crashed against the steel counter—ceramic splintered, coffee pooling in dark rivulets—as Leana seized her radio. She snatched the second response bag and an extra oxygen cylinder, her boots striking the floor as she bolted out alongside Rodrigo. Could this ship ever grant her a moment's peace?

Rodrigo kept pace, the oxygen tank and first response bag thudding against his hip with each stride. Port side flashed by—even numbers, right path, she muttered under her breath, orienting herself in the blur.

Luisa Sorres flung 8136's door wide as Leana charged in first.

Felix lay sprawled across the bed, lips blue, chest jerking in shallow gasps, a sour stench of sweat choking the air. Leana clamped a non-rebreather mask over his face, oxygen hissing, her pulse hammering—save him, now, duty roared. "Pulse?" she snapped, fingers digging into his carotid, faint and fading.

"Erratic," Rodrigo rasped, pulse oximeter flashing 68%, hypoxia's crimson glare. His hands shook, sealing the mask, eyes darting to Felix's still face, a nurse fraying under five years' weight. Leana's radio barked: "Team to 8136—Code Blue, severe distress." She drove an intravenous needle, saline dripping, her jaw tight—could they pull him back?

The intercom blared overhead: "Code Blue team—Stateroom 8136." Leana drove an intravenous needle into Felix's vein, the saline dripping as she secured it with swift, practised tape. Three minutes stretched like wire—Gutierrez stormed in at 6:03 am, stethoscope swinging, his boots a war drum. Mkhwanazi and Roberta followed, gurney clattering, Jit hauling the defibrillator, its cables a tangled lifeline. No Srinivas—Leana's gut knotted, his absence a blade. Roberta's clipped "We've parted ways" flashed, her nod sharp—good riddance, but not now.

"Saturation 68%, 15 litres, no gain," Rodrigo reported, stepping back as Gutierrez pressed his stethoscope, face carved with focus.

"Crackles bilateral—wet lungs. History—now."

"Diabetes, Atrial fibrillation, shortness of breath on exertion," Luisa choked from the corner, tissue shredding, her terror a weight Leana felt in her bones.

Gutierrez's eyes met hers, a steel command: "Leana—airway. Mkhwanazi—meds. Jit—AED. Rodrigo—compressions, go."

A swift response mobilised security, housekeeping, and guest services, each unit acting with precision amidst the unfolding crisis. Security promptly guarded the doorway, ensuring a controlled environment. Rosanna, the guest services manager, escorted Mrs. Sorres from the room with calm authority, clearing the space for the medical team's focus. Housekeeping formed the stretcher team, tasked with lifting, moving, and transporting the patient— remained on standby outside the stateroom. Though not medical personnel, this team had been rigorously trained to manage all distractions, allowing the medical staff to concentrate solely on performing CPR.

Rodrigo knelt, palms slamming Felix's chest, 110 beats a minute, sweat streaking his brow, each thud a plea cracking his calm—hold on, mate.

Leana gripped the bag-valve mask, forcing air, her arms trembling, Felix's blue lips searing her mind—duty screamed fight, but loss loomed, a shadow she couldn't shake. "Srinivas—8136, where are you?" she hissed into the radio, static mocking her. "Bloody useless," she snarled, phone flaring—a metronome app pulsing with Rodrigo's desperate rhythm.

Jit tore AED pads open, razor scraping, her hands curt, eyes avoiding Leana's—old Thailand friction flaring in silence. "Clear—analysing," she barked, voice tight. The AED droned at 6:10 am: "No shock advised. No pulse present, PEW Continue resuscitation." Jit's jaw twitched, strain buried, her rift with Leana a silent thorn.

Gutierrez's fists clenched, sweat beading, his "Adrenaline, 1 milligram, IV, after second cycle" a strained growl. "Roberta, log it,"

JIT quickly instructed to continue CPR for PEA with no pulse.

Gutierrez snapped, taking Rodrigo's place at 6:12 am, his compressions fierce, voice cracking: "Come on, Felix, fight."

Mkhwanazi's syringe flashed, her "Adrenaline in" at 6:13 am steady, but her fingers faltered, a pause as she met Felix's glazed eyes, grief flickering beneath her steel—a nurse's heart bending

Leana pumped air, two breaths per 30 thrusts, Felix's chest barely rising, her mind racing—Luisa's sob, 56 years, could she steal him back? "Equal bilaterally," Rodrigo gasped, fraying, his hands shaking as he steadied the IV. "Hs and Ts—what's killing him?" Gutierrez demanded at 6:14 am, stepping back, Rodrigo surging in, arms pistoning.

"Hyperkalaemia?" Leana ventured, monitor glaring PEA—a death knell. "Diabetes, meds—potassium's likely."

"Plausible," Mkhwanazi murmured, oxygen cylinder steady, her voice soft, eyes distant—Felix slipping too far.

"No jugular distension," Gutierrez countered,

"MI's favourite—enzymes'll tell. Jit—switch."

Jit tagged in at 6:18 am, compressions brutal, her silence heavy, tension coiling with Leana.

"Second adrenaline, 1 milligram," Gutierrez ordered,

Mkhwanazi pushing it at 6:19 am, her breath catching, a sob swallowed.

Srinivas lurched in at 6:20 am, scrubs creased, eyes bruised, ten minutes late.

Leana's glare scorched him. "Where were you? Radio's dead—again."

"No signal—exhaustion," Srinivas muttered, gloves fumbling, shame flickering.

"Rubbish," Leana spat, ventilating harder, Felix's weight crushing her.

"Compressions, Srinivas—now," Gutierrez roared, pointing to Jit's spot.

Srinivas knelt at 6:22 am, hands shaky, then locking under Gutierrez's fire.

"Pulse check," Gutierrez called at 6:24 am, PEA unyielding. Srinivas probed Felix's neck—no pulse, his voice thin: "Nothing."

"Third adrenaline," Gutierrez said, Mkhwanazi's syringe trembling at 6:25 am, her pause longer now, eyes wet, a crack in her calm. Leana's arms burned, mask fogging, Felix's stillness a vice—could duty defy this?

"Rotate—Rodrigo," Gutierrez snapped at 6:27 am, Srinivas slinking back, sweat rivers on his face.

"Fourth adrenaline—6:29 am," Mkhwanazi pushed, voice breaking, her hands slow, grief seeping.

Jit swapped in at 6:31 am, her rhythm fierce but eyes distant, Leana's shadow a weight she dodged.

"Pulse check," Gutierrez rasped at 6:33 am, Rodrigo's fingers on Felix's neck—nothing, his head shaking, shoulders sagging, a man spent.

"Fifth adrenaline—6:34 am," Gutierrez said, voice flint, Mkhwanazi's syringe near dropping, her exhale a shudder, tears held back.

At 6:35 am, Felix's chest lay still, monitor flat, asystole's hum a blade—25 minutes burned. Gutierrez stepped back, fists unclenched, sweat gleaming, his "MI, thrombus—nothing left" a broken whisper, strain carving his face, a doctor defeated. "Call it."

Leana froze, mask locked in her grip, Rodrigo's eyes hollow, staring at the floor. Mkhwanazi's head bowed, a choked breath escaping, her hands still on the empty syringe, grief raw beneath her calm. Jit's compressions stopped, her silence deafening, tension with Leana unspoken. Srinivas shrank against the wall, gaze averted, his delay a ghost. "Time of death, 6:35," Gutierrez said, voice hollow, chart slamming shut.

Leana's phone went dark. She tore off the mask, gloves slick with sweat, and the oxygen hiss died down. Felix's last shudder seared into her bones.

Mkhwanazi coiled the IV, her breath catching, a sob swallowed.

Srinivas shrank back, wiping his brow, dodging her gaze—logs would haunt him later.

Gutierrez stood unbowed, his shadow a jagged lifeline across the bed, the anchor they'd gripped for 25 brutal minutes.

Jit tore the final printout from the machine, a stark, unwavering line etching Felix's end, then yanked the cable free with a faint snap, leaving the pads clinging to his still chest—silent sentinels of a battle lost.

"We battled," he said, voice raw but resolute, locking eyes with Rodrigo, Mkhwanazi, Leana, Jit and Srinivas.

"That's what matters." Luisa's wail shattered free, a jagged blade in the hush, and Gutierrez turned to it, duty shifting once more.

Leana's throat seized, stylus scratching into the tablet—68% oxygen saturation, PEA, suspected MI. Her hand hovered, as Luisa crumpled against the wall, nails raking her face, her cry a wound Leana felt in her gut. Her boots scraped the carpet, instinct tugging her near, but Gutierrez's raised hand stopped her—his burden now.

At 6:40 am, Gutierrez stepped into the corridor, his voice a low murmur against Deck 8's hum where Mrs Sorres was sitting with Rosanna the guest services manager. "Mrs. Sorres, I'm so sorry—Felix has passed."

Luisa's sob split the air, sharp as splintered glass, and he steadied her to a chair, his shadow a quiet fortress beside her breaking form. Leana caught the sound through the cracked door, a shard sinking deep.

Inside 8136, Leana draped a sheet over Felix, its crisp edge trembling in her grip, as the cabin's stagnant air thickened with loss. Roberta carried the medical bags out, its clatter a dull requiem, Mkhwanazi trailing with the rubbish—needles, wrappers, a spent adrenaline vial rattling in the red bag. Jit lingered near the door, pen scraping notes, her silence a jagged thorn under Leana's skin. That old friction from Thailand—triage clash, Jit's curt "Yes, Lead"—simmered still, her quiet now biting just as deep.

"Srinivas," Leana said, her voice level as he turned, fumbling with his stethoscope. "Check my phone and radio—something's amiss, I'm telling you."

"IT logs don't deceive," she snapped, pinning his gaze until he flinched first, slinking out. Gutierrez caught her eye from the corridor—a fleeting nod of accord, then gone. She'd flagged Srinivas's radio lapses before—each evasion a fracture in their chain. Today, it stole minutes. Perhaps a life.

At 07h00 am, Felix's gurney rumbled through Deck 0's hush, security carving a path, guests ushered aside with brisk apologies. Leana steadied the foot, the sheet fluttering white—a shroud for a battle lost. At the medical centre, In the morgue's icy grip, she unzipped the body bag, steel chilling her gloved hands, Felix's face slack—blue faded to ash. A man who'd climbed stairs and faltered forever.

Luisa shuffled in behind Rosanna, fingers grazing his cheek, whispers drowning in the refrigeration's drone — "Fifty-six years, my love…" Leana stepped back, breath clouding her chest a vice around an anniversary she couldn't salvage. Rosanna eased Luisa out after ten minutes, her sobs ricocheting down the hall. Leana re-zipped the bag, the zip's rasp a final knell, and locked the morgue door.

Back at the nurses' station, she slumped into a chair, tablet glowing with the maritime death form—time, medications, vitals. Rodrigo slid in beside her, his pen scratching the incident report, last shift's wear etched beneath his eyes.

"You bearing up?" he asked, voice soft, a lifeline through the gloom.

Her pen stalled, ink bleeding into the margin. "Must," she said, jaw locked. "Your final call—a brutal farewell."

His grin flickered, faint but alive. "Better than sunburns." He tapped the wrapped box on the desk—team gift, still sealed. "I'll miss this madness."

"The madness will miss you," she replied, nudging his shoulder. "Keep that heart ticking ashore."

"Done," he chuckled, low and warm, a salve against Felix's ghost.

The clinic opened at 8:00 a.m., Bahamian sun glaring through the porthole, a queue already coiling—sunburnt shoulders from yesterday, a sprained ankle, a child's earache piercing the air.

Leana taped gauze, checked vitals, Felix's flatline a shadow clawing her edges. Gutierrez leaned on the counter, coffee cooling, watching her hands weave precision from a decade's scars.

"Tough one," he said, voice gravel against the BP cuff's hum.

"You held us steady—kept the rails firm," she said, snapping a chart shut, Felix's blue lips flashing unbidden.

"Luisa's eyes—those stay," he murmured, sipping slow, steam curling. "Rodrigo's send-off's tonight—steakhouse, 6:00. He's earned it."

"Wouldn't miss it," she said, a grin breaking through the weight, her first full breath since 6:35 am.

The day dragged on—Leana's voice held firm, guiding Mkhwanazi through a suture on a deckhand's torn palm, the needle flashing silver in the clinic's stark light. "Tighter stitches—less scarring," she said, Mkhwanazi nodding swift, her focus a blade's edge.

The day dragged on—Leana's voice held firm, guiding Mkhwanazi through a suture on a deckhand's torn palm, the needle flashing silver in the clinic's stark light. "Tighter stitches—less scarring," she said, Mkhwanazi nodding swift, her focus a blade's edge.

Roberta delivered Felix's lab results—cardiac enzymes soaring, Pro-BNP off the charts. Heart failure, likely myocardial infarction. possible embolism, the dyspnoea matched. Leana filed it, the cold data a slap against Luisa's raw wail. She'd called it—a fleeting triumph, hollow as ash.

By 4:00 p.m., the clinic quieted, sunburns giving way to paperwork's grind. Jared Simpson, the port agent, breezed in—dreadlocks swaying, voice lilting as he dumped a sheaf of forms. "Bahamian officials cleared the ship—Felix's repatriation's sorted," he said, his grin a fleeting spark. "Ever dived the Lucayan caves? Six miles of tunnels—pirates bled there, limestone jaws clamping shut."

Leana's pen stilled, her gaze lifting. "No chance this trip."

"Next run," he winked, snagging Felix's passport copy from Rosanna. "Got you cleared quick—owe me a rum."

"Agreed," she said, a half-smile cracking the day's weight, his banter a fleeting lifeline.

At 5:00 PM, Dr Gutierrez and Leana convened to deliberate over whether to proceed with Rodrigo's farewell dinner in the wake of Felix's tragic passing, a loss that weighed heavily on their hearts. Leana, her voice tinged with sorrow, acknowledged the day's profound hardship for the entire team, suggesting that coming together might offer solace and strength. She urged, with quiet resolve, that the dinner should not be cancelled, believing it could foster unity amidst their grief.

At 6:00 pm, the steakhouse glowed amber, lanterns swaying over the crew's table, Deck 5's hum muted beyond the glass. Leana slid into a seat, the sear of meat and beer's bite cutting through the air—a jagged shift from antiseptic's sting. Gutierrez hoisted his glass, voice thundering over the clink. "To Rodrigo—five years, the finest nurse we've known. Fair winds, mate."

"Cheers!" Glasses collided, foam spilling across the wood. Leana pushed the slim gift over—team gift, etched "R.G. 2020-2025"—her fingers grazing his.

He ripped it open, grin splitting wide, the watch gleaming under the warm light. "You lot—this is too much, a G-watch" he said, voice thick, tracing the inscription. "Thank you."

"Learnt from you," Leana said, locking eyes, her throat snagging. "That first code—you kept us steady."

"Couldn't let the greenhorn flounder," he fired back, clapping her shoulder, his laugh a warm balm.

Jit sat silent, nursing a beer, her gaze darting to Leana then dropping—same edge, same rift.

"Jit," Leana said, voice low over the din. "Medication counts tally?"

"Always," Jit replied, curt, eyes fixed down. Twelve years, and that barb still pricked.

Following dinner, the medical team gathered in the Eleanor Atrium at 7:30 p.m., seeking a moment's respite beneath its gilded elegance, where the space unfurled in a symphony of opulence. Crystal chandeliers cast a warm, amber glow across the polished marble floors, their light dancing on the deep claret curtains that framed towering windows overlooking the endless sea. At the atrium's heart stood a regal portrait of Queen Eleanor, her stern yet compassionate gaze seeming to watch over the gathering, a silent sentinel of the ship's legacy. The violinists' gentle strains filled the air, their melodies a soft balm against the day's raw wounds, weaving through the room's rich tapestry of velvet seating and intricate gold filigree. Leana sat between Mkhwanazi and Dr Gutierrez, her shoulders loosening as the music dulled the sharp edge of grief that had lingered since Felix's passing—a loss that still pressed a tender ache into her chest. Gutierrez's quiet nod, weathered hands folded, showed his team's resilience; meanwhile, Srinivas, next to Roberta, shifted impatiently, wanting to escape. Rodrigo, Roberta and Jit shared a quiet exchange nearby, their presence a grounding comfort that underscored the bond uniting the team, forged through shared sorrow and unwavering resolve.

As the music swelled, the violinists paused to honour the medical team, their words prompting the seated crowd to stand and applaud—a wave of respect that warmed Leana's weary heart, catching her off guard. Under Queen Eleanor's watchful gaze, this recognition, after a day shadowed by such profound loss, lifted the team's spirits, weaving a fragile thread of solace through their mourning, a poignant testament to their strength together.

At 9:30 pm, Leana trudged wearily back to her cabin, her boots echoing with a heavy thud against Deck 0's cold steel floor, the faint glow of Freeport's lights receding through the porthole as the ship pressed on into the night. Jared's tales of cave explorations lingered in her thoughts—six miles of shadowed depths, a realm beyond her reach on this voyage, a fleeting distraction from the day's weight. Her bunk creaked under her as she collapsed, the ship's low, rhythmic drone a subdued lullaby that failed to quiet her restless mind. Images swirled relentlessly: Felix's blue lips during his final moments, Srinivas's evasive avoidance after his errors, Jit's piercing glare of frustration. Yet, amidst the turmoil, the memory of the crowd's heartfelt appreciation in the Eleanor Atrium for the team's tireless efforts offered a glimmer of solace, easing the ache in her chest and reminding her of the lives they had touched, even on such a harrowing day.

The tablet's screen flared to life, an email from IT flashing with stark clarity: "Unable to retrieve logs for Dr. Srinivas—router missing, presumed stolen."

Leana's brow creased deeply, a bitter unease coiling within her stomach. Who would pilfer a router? The realisation dawned that she must now offer Srinivas an apology, her earlier accusation—"No logs, no proof"—fading into insignificance. Roberta's declaration, "We've parted ways," accompanied by her silent, approving nod of farewell, lingered vividly—yet a troubling suspicion emerged: had Srinivas taken it to conceal his actions? The notion gnawed at her, relentless and piercing, rekindling the pain of his absence during Felix's critical code. A further doubt surfaced: without a signal, how had he known to respond? Resolved, she determined to confront him the following day.

As New York's silhouette loomed on the horizon, heralding a new nurse and fresh challenges, Leana massaged her tense neck, feeling Felix's burden gradually ease, Luisa's anguished sob lingering as a faint, indelible mark. They had battled for twenty-five minutes, each breath a fierce struggle against the encroaching void—a resolve that anchored her still. Exhaustion finally claimed her, the ship's gentle, rhythmic sway cradling her into sleep as dawn approached.

Chapter Seven: Last Sea Day

Leana's boots came to a halt on deck at 08:00 am, stuck in place by an unshakable weight. She'd watched the amber sunrise bleed across the waves, its warm glow glinting like molten gold, but it couldn't pierce the heaviness clawing her chest. Felix and Luisa—fifty-six years woven tight—unravelled on this cursed cruise, their love snuffed out in a sterile cabin. The thought gnawed raw, a wound too fresh after 25 minutes of clawing him back, only to lose.

Luisa had wandered alone that final day aboard the Majestic Voyager, her frail frame chasing ghosts of their cherished bond through the ship's gleaming corridors. Every death here was a stain—grief seeping into the holidaymakers' joy, a bitter smear Leana couldn't scrub clean. Fifty-six years, and it ended in her hands. Tears stung hot down her cheeks as she turned from the view, the salt air biting as she retreated inside.

She dialled Rodrigo's phone, stepping into the medical centre's stark light. "We'll see you at the crew bar tonight—your final send-off. Take the day, but if an emergency hits, I might need you."

"Thank you, Leana," Rodrigo replied, his voice a mix of warmth and weariness. "Hard to fathom it's my last. I keep seeing Mr. Sorres—us, the last ones with him. I whisper a prayer for him, for Luisa. May he rest easy now."

"Time races when we're snatching lives, doesn't it?" she said, forcing a grin through the ache. "Tonight, we'll toast you proper—and a quiet prayer for Felix."

As she tackled her morning tasks, a quiet melancholy clung like damp fog. Rodrigo's departure would gouge the team—he'd been her rock, unlike Srinivas, whose radio logs still taunted her with Deck 8's ping. Jit's silent barbs lingered too, fraying the edges. She prayed his replacement would match his steel, not buckle under the strain.

Rosanna's call cut through her haze, the guest services manager's voice crisp. "Leana, I'm sorting Felix Sorres' funeral arrangements. Could you meet me in my office to finalise?"

"Of course, Rosanna. I'll be there shortly," Leana replied, her tone hardening with resolve. Felix's family deserved every ounce of care she could muster—duty over despair.

Her boots echoed toward Rosanna's office, thoughts swirling through the week's relentless trials—diverse patients, unpredictable ailments, a crucible of adaptation and endurance. Felix's blue lips flashed, Srinivas's dodge, Jit's glare—all testing her marrow.

"Come in," Rosanna beckoned at her knock. The office gleamed, orderly as her meticulous mind, a stark contrast to the chaos Leana carried. Rosanna waved her to a seat. "I've liaised with a New York funeral home for Felix Sorres. Customs and Border Protection are informed; the coroner boards at docking to examine him—likely with questions. Ensure your team's ready. His children arrive to collect him. Review these documents—everything must be spot-on."

Leana pored over the papers, her stylus tracing every line—times, medications, vitals—her chest tight with the burden to shield Felix's kin. "It's all in order, Rosanna," she said, voice steady. "Thank you for managing this so well. It eases me, knowing they'll be looked after."

Rosanna's nod was grave, her eyes glistening. "It's the least we can offer them," she said, her voice thick with a sorrow that mirrored Leana's own.

Leana stepped from the office, her boots scuffing the corridor's gleam, thoughts snagging on Rodrigo and the farewell looming that evening. It'd be a raw affair—tears and laughter tangled tight—but vital, a chance to honour his steady hand through five years of chaos, to send him off with the fire he deserved. She drew a sharp breath, steeling herself to carve a day worth remembering for him, for the team still reeling from Felix's loss.

Back at the medical centre, Leana discussed the stolen router with Dr. Gutierrez, who advised her to hold off on the matter until tomorrow's meeting. "Let's not overshadow Rodrigo's final send-off today," Gutierrez said, her tone firm yet considerate.

Leana watched as Mkhwanazi prepped the morning clinic, a quiet melancholy seeping into her chest, heavy as the dawn's grey pallor. Zhao's frail form shuffled in— eighty years etched into her delicate bones—and Leana's voice softened. "Good morning, Zhao. How can I assist you today?"

"Call me Zhao, please," she murmured, her face pale, drawn tight with weariness. "Swallowing's been a battle these past two years. My doctor said soft foods, solids if I can bear them."

Mkhwanazi leaned in, her gaze sharp yet gentle, as Zhao unravelled her tale—nausea gnawing constantly, muscles aching deep, though her bowels held steady, no fever, no pain, no motion sickness plaguing her with dizziness or headaches. "Have you tried anything for relief?" Mkhwanazi asked, concern carving lines into her brow.

Zhao shook her head, resolute. "No medications, if I can avoid them. Just intravenous fluids and dextrose, please."

"Of course. Let's settle you in—Dr. Gutierrez will assess you first," Mkhwanazi replied, her smile a quiet anchor.

Gutierrez pored over Zhao's chart, his brow furrowing as the details sank in—a petite woman, grey hair framing a face of quiet defiance, her low BMI a stark note against her resilience. He approached, his voice measured. "Zhao, I'm Dr. Gutierrez. Two years struggling to swallow— that's a heavy load. I'd suggest anti-emetics for the nausea, but the fluids and dextrose alone won't sustain you properly."

"Thank you, Doctor," Zhao said, her tone weary yet warm. "I'd take the anti-emetics. I know the fluids aren't enough, but they'll carry me to my doctor. Could you draw blood for sodium and potassium levels?"

Leana lingered nearby, her hands itching to act, Felix's blue lips flickering unbidden. Zhao's fight stirred her—another soul clinging on, like they'd tried with Felix. She'd see this through, for Rodrigo's last day, for the team still frayed.

"Of course," Dr. Gutierrez said, his voice laced with quiet admiration for Zhao's grasp of her own frail state. "Nurse Mkhwanazi, prepare a litre of Ringer's lactate for Zhao, with 100 millilitres of 5% dextrose, as she's requested."

Leana craved a distraction—anything to mute Felix's flatline still ringing in her skull—and seized control, her hands deft as she pierced Zhao's vein with a steady jab, securing vascular access. Crimson welled in the vial as she drew blood, then she hooked up the fluids, the dextrose saline dripping like a fragile thread of hope. Her mind slipped to Rodrigo—those bloodshot eyes, rum-soaked from wild nights, a reckless gleam she'd never begrudged. Not when he'd been her anchor, steady through every storm. She glanced at Zhao, her eyes fluttering shut, relief easing the taut lines of her face as the fluids wove their subtle spell—a fleeting triumph slicing through a day still jagged with loss.

"Thank you," Zhao murmured, her voice a soft echo of gratitude.

"You're welcome, Zhao," Leana replied, her chest swelling with a flicker of pride. "Glad we could ease you."

"Thank you for indulging me, Dr. Gutierrez," Zhao added, her gaze locking his with weary sincerity.

Gutierrez studied her as she rested on the bed, a shiver rippling through her slight frame, her eyes drifting closed. The medical equipment's low hum filled the silence, a steady pulse beneath his concern. "Zhao," he said, voice gentle yet firm, "I see you need strength to disembark tomorrow for your doctor, but we must dig deeper—find what's driving this."

"Certainly," she answered, faint but resolute. "But I know my limits—this will hold me for now."

Mkhwanazi stepped in, the basic metabolic panel rustling in her hands. Gutierrez scanned it, his brow creasing as Zhao's potassium spiked at 6.3—everything else steady, normal. "Zhao, your potassium's elevated," he said, urgency threading his tone. "Hyperkalaemia's unlikely with your history—could be haemolysis skewing it. I'd like to redraw the blood."

"Do an ECG first—check the T waves," Zhao countered, her eyes snapping open, fixed on him with a doctor's steel.

Gutierrez blinked, surprised. "Are you a physician?"

She paused, then nodded. "Retired—years ago."

His respect sharpened, a nod acknowledging her clarity, her command. She was no mere patient—she knew the stakes. He flicked his gaze to Leana, already prepping the ECG, her hands steady despite the ache of Felix's ghost. "Very well, Dr. Zhao," he said, voice firm. "ECG first, then we'll move forward." She dipped her head, a faint approval in her tired eyes.

Leana's hands moved with quiet precision as she fixed the ECG electrodes to Dr. Zhao's chest, each wire a tether to answers she craved—something to drown Felix's flatline still haunting her skull.

Dr. Gutierrez watched, his mind wrestling the thin line between Zhao's will and his duty, a balance he hoped they'd strike together. She'd leave the Majestic Voyager stronger—he'd see to it, her resolve sparking a flicker of his own.

"Retired, you say?" Gutierrez said, a wry smile tugging his lips as he caught Leana's eye. "Then let's get you back on your feet, Doctor."

"Very well, Dr. Zhao," he continued, his gaze tracing the ECG printout as it spooled out, sharp lines etching secrets. "We've got pathological anterior Q waves here—hints of an old heart attack. Can you shed light on this?"

Zhao's brow creased, her frail hands tightening briefly. "The last casualty visit, they said my ECG was normal—called it heartburn. But years back, one showed premature beats."

"Curious," Gutierrez murmured, thumb grazing his chin as he studied the strip. "No premature beats now, though." His respect deepened—a fellow healer, her grit mirroring his own fire for the craft, even as Leana's steady hands grounded the moment.

Gutierrez's brow tightened as he pored over the printout, peaked T waves spiking in V3 and V4, variables nagging in V5 and V6. The rhythm held normal, but those peaks gnawed at him. He glanced at Zhao, her face a mask of calm over a flicker of dread.

"Dr. Zhao," he said, voice soft yet edged with steel, "your expertise is clear, but we must pool it with ours. These findings—we can't dismiss other causes without more tests."

Her eyes met his, a storm of trust and trepidation swirling there. She knew her limits had frayed—her health now rested with them, with him. "Proceed, then," she whispered, the words a fragile surrender.

"Dr. Zhao," he said, voice cautious, "these T wave abnormalities—we need to unpack them."

"Certainly," she replied, her tone even, though a tremor betrayed her.

"I'd suggest halting the Ringer's lactate," Zhao said, her gaze locked on the printout, "and switching to dextrose saline, over two hours. It'll suit me better now."

"Agreed," Gutierrez replied, nodding briskly. "Leana, adjust it."

But unease coiled in his gut—something lurked beneath. "Dr. Zhao, I'd strongly recommend further tests—a full blood count, at least—to rule out other culprits

Dr. Zhao faltered, her frail frame tensing, fingers brushing the jade pendant at her neck—a habit, Leana noted, from days steeped in Chinese tradition. She drew a deep breath, steadying her resolve.

"No, thank you, Dr. Gutierrez," she said, voice firm despite the weariness etching her eyes. "Fluids will do for now. My family always leaned on balance—less intrusion, let the body find its way."

Gutierrez's chest tightened, his mind snagging on Felix's blue lips—another loss if he failed to act. Zhao's clarity, her doctor's steel, demanded respect, but what if her choice hid a ticking bomb? Duty screamed for tests, yet forcing her risked shattering trust, her dignity. "Are you certain?" he pressed, concern carving deep lines across his brow. "These tests could catch something critical."

Her gaze locked his, unyielding yet soft, like bamboo bending but unbroken. "I grasp the risks, Doctor—I'm choosing knowingly. It's my way—rooted in years of learning, not just medicine, but how we heal back home. I'll sign your 'against medical advice' form if you need it."

Leana caught the weight in her words, a glimpse of a world where trust in nature's rhythm outran sterile probes—a choice she'd seen clash with Western haste before.

Gutierrez nodded, jaw tight, swallowing the urge to argue—her right trumped his fear, but the weight of letting go clung like damp steel.

The fluids finished in just over an hour, and Zhao rose, discharged, her steps firm despite the exhaustion Leana knew must claw at her bones.

"Take care, Dr. Zhao," Leana called, her voice soft as the retired physician strode from the medical centre, a quiet strength masking the ordeal's toll.

"Thank you all," Zhao replied, pausing to dip her head at each of them—Gutierrez, Mkhwanazi, Leana—before vanishing beyond the door.

The air shifted as it closed, tension bleeding out like mist, Mkhwanazi's sigh a faint release as sweat glistened on her brow. "That was intense," Gutierrez muttered, kneading the back of his neck, his gaze sweeping the team. "Never treated someone so sharp about their own state."

"Truly," Leana said, her eyes distant, Felix's blue lips flashing unbidden. "I just pray she reaches her doctor tomorrow."

"Same," Mkhwanazi added, her warm tone edged with worry, shaking off the unease to tackle the cleaning ahead.

"I need to sort the orientation pack for the new nurse," Leana said, her voice steadying. "His first weeks will test us all."

"Smart move," Gutierrez replied, a faint smile breaking through. "He'll lean on your steadiness."

All day, Leana immersed herself in work, losing track of time until Roberta's gentle tap signaled the clinic's closing. Roberta delivered a patient update, her voice steady yet warm. "Leana, Marian not only completed her intravenous antibiotics but also posted a glowing TripAdvisor review: 'The Majestic Voyager's medical team outshines any land hospital!' Moving down the list, Robyn's mobility has significantly improved, Sara's cast is still perfectly intact, and Celeste's anaphylaxis follow-up shows no complications." With precise, practiced movements, Roberta assembled their discharge packets, each final bill neatly clipped to crisp medical records. Another voyage's cases closed, another set of lives touched.

Leana's eyes sparkled with gratitude. "Roberta, your talent is unmatched—you're truly the heart of this operation, keeping everything together from the shadows." My deepest thanks for your unwavering dedication.

That evening, Leana sat alone in the medical centre's stillness, paperwork scattered like debris across the desk, each note slotted with care into the orientation pack. Zhao's quiet defiance hung in her mind—thoughts over Felix's ghost—yet the new nurse loomed, another shift, another battle to keep the line from fraying.

"Leana, still here?" Mkhwanazi's voice broke the hush, warm as a lantern's glow.

"Yes," Leana replied, a faint smile tugging her lips. "Just finishing the pack for the new nurse."

"Let me lend a hand," Mkhwanazi offered, her smile a balm that eased the ache in Leana's chest. Together, they sifted through documents and guidelines, a steady rhythm weaving between them, a silent bond stitching the night's edges.

"He'll need to pick up quick," Leana murmured, her gaze tracing the tidy files. "It's a steep climb ahead."

"Change bites hard," Mkhwanazi said, her voice soft yet firm. "But we'll guide him through."

Leana nodded, a swell of gratitude warming her—Rodrigo's steadiness echoed in Mkhwanazi's resolve, a lifeline against Srinivas's shadow. The days would test them, but this—this unspoken unity—held stronger than any plan she could muster.

The crew bar thrummed with murmurs and the clatter of cutlery, the medical team crowded around a broad table, the air thick with revelry. It brimmed to the rafters—some dubbed it a party's pulse, others a last hurrah before sign-off.

"Alright, everyone," Dr. Gutierrez boomed, hoisting his glass. "To Nurse Rodrigo—our bedrock, our mate. We'll feel your absence keenly."

"Hear, hear!" the team chorused, glasses clashing with a bright ring. Leana's smile warmed toward Rodrigo, tears pricking her eyes, unshed but heavy.

"Thank you, all," Rodrigo said, voice rough with feeling. "You've been my world."

Leana leaned close, pressing a drink into his hand. "I'll miss those rum-red eyes," she murmured

Gutierrez clapped Rodrigo's back. "A privilege, Nurse Rodrigo. Our paths'll cross again."

"Here's to it," Rodrigo replied, lifting his glass anew.

Laughter swelled as the night unfurled, memories spilling out—sharp jabs and soft recalls. Srinivas, Jit, and Roberta traded tales of Rodrigo's grit, their words weaving a tapestry of his mark on them, warm as the bar's amber glow.

Leana drew Srinivas aside, her voice low. "About the radio—I'm sorry. We're digging into the stolen router." His eyes flickered, a shadow of unease at "digging," but he nodded, muted.

She raised her glass to him, a wry edge cutting through. "Here's hoping the new nurse keeps up with your late-night charm."

The team spilled into the dance floor's throng, voices and steps syncing to the beat, infectious and fierce. Leana swayed, a rare unity pulsing through her—a lifeline against Rodrigo's void, the 25-minute fight for Felix still raw.

"Rodrigo, you're unmatched!" Srinivas bellowed, barely piercing the din.

"Stay well, mate!" Mkhwanazi grinned, her light unwavering.

The farewell roared on, a testament to their bond, and though Leana felt the sting of goodbye, those shared moments burned bright—a torch for the storms ahead.

Then Jit's phone shattered the din, frantic and shrill. Ni Luh's voice trembled through—gut pain stabbing, urination relentless, constipation gripping, hard stools passed earlier.

Jit muttered apologies, bolting for the medical centre, Srinivas trailing swift behind.

Leana watched Jit and Srinivas vanish out of the crew bar, her gut twisting—another test, another tug at the fraying line. The bar's roar faded behind her as she turned away, boots heavy on Deck 0's steel.

Homeport loomed tomorrow—inventory, new sign-ons, and the authorities circling Felix's death. She'd call it a night, save her strength for the storm ahead.

Jit and Srinivas slipped back from the medical centre, shadows slicing the corridor's buzz, relief a thin shield in Leana's chest.

"Nothing major?" she called, voice taut, holding steady.

"UTI," Jit said, nod sharp, eyes clear of venom.

Ni Luh's chart flashed—'Burning and pain when passing urine,' she'd said, wincing.

Srinivas shrugged, "Urinary tract infection—no fuss," skipping the pelvic, his pen already elsewhere. Leana's gut twisted—too quick. Srinivas's eyes dodged, router's shadow heavy.

Chapter eight: Back to Home port

The Majestic Voyager slid into New York's harbour at 7:00 am, dawn's haze parting for Manhattan's jagged towers, a steel pulse against the pale sky. Leana Ria gripped Deck 12's railing, coffee bitter in her hands, the Statue of Liberty's torch a faint glow. Salt air bit her cheeks, sharp as the homeport's churn—fifteen years at sea, twelve as lead nurse, and still endings stung Felix's blue lips, a fresh scar.

"Guests, we've docked," the intercom blared, gulls drowning its echo. "Disembarkation begins—safe travels." Leana drained her mug, grounds settling like the voyage's weight. Two hours to clear 3,200 souls, scour decks, and brace for new blood—housekeeping buckling, medical teetering with Felix's loss, Ni Luh's crisis, a new nurse to shape.

Deck 0's medical centre hummed at 7:30 am with the housekeeping team, cleaning toilets, wiping down the walls and counters, and mopping the floors. Leana entered and Shamik's folder was ready for the Western Caribbean run. Leana traced his name—Durban RN, five years' steel. Her Cape Town roots stirred—close enough to hope he'd match Rodrigo's grit.

Himanshu Raja loomed in the doorway, security badge glinting, trailed by the coroner, CBP officers, and NYPD's Kevlar bulk. "Leana—They're here for Felix's rundown. Need Gutiérrez too."

She stood, scrubs crisp. "Morning, Himanshu. Gentlemen."

She dialled. "Dr. Gutiérrez, Coroners here."

.

His "On it" snapped back, steady.

Gutierrez marched in at 6:45, jaw set, Freeport's weight heavy—Luisa's sob still sharp. "Felix Sorres—myocardial infarction, acute thrombus sealed it," he said, voice clipped, charting 68% oxygen, five adrenaline rounds, pulseless activity unyielding. The coroner unzipped the morgue bag, pen scrawling "natural causes." CBP handed documents to Himanshu, NYPD murmuring clearance. Leana logged it, Felix's blue lips a stone in her ribs—his last gasp, their fight, gone.

"Leana!" Melissa Cleaver burst in, HR's clipboard rattling. "Shamik's running late—he missed the shuttle. Just called to say they left without him. I notified the port agent."

Leana stepped out with Melissa as the gangway thrummed—duffel bags thudded, chatter rose, a dozen languages colliding in the morning air. Near immigration, she caught Rodrigo leaning against a railing, his jeans frayed, eyes rum-red from last night's farewells, the glint of his G-Watch marking time like a silent promise. She pulled him into a hug, his familiar frame anchoring five years of coded emergencies and one week of shared laughter.

"Stay fierce, Rodrigo," she said, her voice catching, her sleeve brushing away tears before they could fall.

"Family, boss," he rasped, his grin warm but eyes glistening under the terminal's harsh lights. "Don't forget." He slung his bag over his shoulder and melted into the JFK-bound crowd. Leana watched until he disappeared, the space where he'd stood now hollow, his steady presence already a ghost.

At 08:00, Mkhwanazi's voice cut through the medical centre's hum, sharp as a scalpel.

"Leana—Ni Luh's at Queens Hospital. Pregnant, haemorrhaging—collapsed in the airport toilets. Ambulance took her; port agent's scrambling for a referral letter."

Leana's boots rooted to the floor. Last night's chart flashed in her mind—UTI., Srinivas's hurried "stable" scribbled in the margins. She snatched the file, her eyes racing over the notes: burning on urination, leukocytes and trace blood, no pelvic exam documented.

"Jit—did Srinivas conduct a visual pelvic exam?" Jit's arms dropped, her stammer quick, eyes on the deck. "No— just the sample. Showed leukocytes, trace blood, but no particles of blood found in urine… UTI, he reckoned. Sent her off., she is going home today,"

"Twelve years here, Jit, and you let him skip that?" Leana's voice cracked, fury burning her throat as she dialled Gutierrez, pacing by the porthole—forklifts droning, blind to their chaos.

Gutierrez's sigh hissed. "Srinivas?"

"Out sightseeing," Leana said.

"Negligence—again," he growled. "Letter's drafting—
. Meeting tonight—he's done dodging."

"Roberta was on the phone with the port agent, and he
stated that Ni Luh is fine. They evaluated her and her bay
seems to be okay, and they are awaiting her referral and
documents."

"Thank you, Roberta, you are the best," Leana said

Gutierrez stepped from his office, referral in hand, his
nod firm, eyes shadowed—ten years in trauma wards,
swapped for cruises to guard his son, Ni Luh's scare
stirring ER ghosts. "Tough lass," he growled, voice gravel,
passing the referral to Roberta. "Thanks for keeping our
admin tight—kept her transfer smooth."

Guests started trickling into the medical centre, the
gangway's hum seeping through steel, New York's salt air
sharp against antiseptic's sting. Roberta stood at the desk,
files stacked neat—Jason's clonidine notes, Celeste's
anaphylaxis chart, Robyn's knee injury.

"Robyn's security report's ready, Leana," she said,
voice calm, radio clipped, handing over Jason's notes.
Leana passed them out, charts heavy—Felix's loss, Ni
Luh's scare, Jerry's glare—a voyage scarred, a shadow
looming for the 5:00 pm meeting.

Jason Roberts came first, arm in arm with Jennifer, his steps steady, face brighter—$1200 bill, clonidine holding, relapse tamed.

"Leana, you pulled me through," he said, voice warm, gratitude raw. Jennifer's eyes stayed hard, her "Thank you" clipped, debt's sting lingering.

Leana's anxiety mounted—her success in caring for someone was undermined by a faltering trust, a situation mirroring Jason's difficult battle against Srinivas's error concerning Ni Luh.

Roberta's nod was soft, her file hand-off seamless, duty a quiet anchor.

Celeste followed, breathing better and showing her epi pen, Jamie's arm firm—$550—life saved. "You're a star, Leana," Celeste said, warmth cutting through.

Jamie's jaw softened, his "Sorry—thanks for everything" low, a crack in his earlier snap. Leana's guilt eased—care held, costs still a bit,

Roberta's steady stack keeping chaos at bay.

Robyn Mathers rolled in, wheelchair creaking, left knee braced, Deck 9's fall a raw mark—$560, X-rays, security report.

Sara Gough followed, her own chair scraping, right ankle cast from tender boat operations—$1,400, mirroring Robyn's fight. They swapped tales, voices low, accidents binding them—Robyn's bar, Sara's slip, company lapses, both. "Need my X-rays, security report," Robyn said, eyes steel, solicitor waiting. Sara nodded, "Same—lawyer's ready."

Leana handed them over, voice firm: "Follow up with your shoreside physician—possibly, physio after." Her gut twisted—care saved their legs, but negligence burned, their bills a debt the ship shirked.

Roberta's "Copies queued" was crisp, her admin grip ensuring their fight could land.

Dr. Zhao and Marian arrived last. Zhao, her jade pendant glinting—$375, dehydration notes. "Best care I've had," she said, voice clear, glancing at Robyn and Sara, a nod to Leana's team—Mkhwanazi's warmth, Gutierrez's steel.

. Robyn's jaw tightened, Sara's voice sharp. "Care's fine—why pay for their ship's fault?"

Zhao's gaze flicked away, her exit swift, no answer for their fire.

Finally, Marian collected her notes and bill. Roberta and Leana warmly thanked her for the glowing TripAdvisor review. Marian beamed, saying, "Without you all, I wouldn't have enjoyed this cruise. You went far beyond medical care to make this trip truly memorable."

Leana's throat caught—duty shone, trust cracked, costs a blade no care could dull.

"Jit—stocks good?" Leana probed, while shredding old logs.

"Always," Jit clipped, pen stabbing logs.

Leana let it lie—tonight would shift it.

At noon Roberta provided an update, Ni Luh's labs showed infection driven urinary tract infection. Foetus intact. She is admitted for observation.
. Leana exhaled , guilt a blade—Srinivas's rush, her trust, cost a life. Care trumped haste, etched deep.

Shamik arrived at 2 pm, boots dusty, Durban drawl thick.

"Hello, I am looking for Leana, the Lead nurse"

Leana was at the nurses' station and she saw him. He looked to be like he was between 25-30 years old, but his actual age was forty. He had a face that was difficult to read. His voice was strong and commanding and had great pronunciation of the English dialect. He had black hair, brown eyes and a light beard and a moustache. He stood firm, upright and had light brown eyes that look tired and was wondering if she had another Rodrigo

"I'm Leana Ria, and I'm truly relieved to meet you," she said, extending her hand. His grip was firm, his smile tentative, and his eyes scanned the corridor as if seeking something familiar.

"I'm Shamik. Many call me Sham or Shammy—whichever you prefer," he replied, his voice warm but edged with uncertainty.

"I understand you had some difficulties with transport this morning," Leana said, guiding him through the ship's polished hallways, the faint hum of engines vibrating beneath their feet.

Shamik gave a wry smile. "Yes, I missed the bus, the safety briefing, orientation, and lunch—everything, it seems."

Nurse Mkhwanazi, following with a gentle smile, chimed in, "Typical Durbanite, perhaps enjoying New York a bit too much?"

Shamik's expression softened, a spark of recognition in his eyes. "You're South African too? That's wonderful."

"Mkhwanazi, born in Johannesburg," she said, her tone friendly.

Leana spoke up, her voice calm but purposeful. "Shammy, you can change, and we'll begin your shift shortly. We'll cover your orientation as we go—welcome to your home for the next six months."

Shamik blinked, startled. "I'm starting now. I had hoped to explore the ship first, perhaps admire the scenery." The floor pulsed slightly, and he glanced around. "Are we departing already?"

Leana's lips curved into a knowing smile as they walked. "Did you think this was a holiday? Our work is exhilarating, but it demands everything. We're preparing for a seven-day cruise, and you're part of it now." Beyond the portholes, the dock was gliding out of view, the ship easing into motion.

They reached his cabin, a modest space three doors from hers. His luggage sat neatly inside, a quiet reminder of the life he'd brought aboard. Shamik set his bag down, exhaling. "I hadn't expected to begin work immediately."

Leana paused in the doorway, her tone measured but carrying a weight of experience. "Let me be clear, Shamik. This job is thrilling, but it's relentless. We work every day—no weekends, no respite. As medical staff, we handle everything from minor ailments to emergencies, all while maintaining a courteous demeanour for passengers, even under pressure. The crew comes from countless countries, which can be enriching, yet it sometimes leads to misunderstandings. We're fortunate; our role grants privileges like access to guest areas and time to explore ports when schedules allow. Others, like housekeeping, rarely get such chances. But it's exhausting—physically, mentally. The pace can push you to your limits, and burnout is a real risk."

Shamik tilted his head, his expression curious but guarded. "That sounds intense, Leana. Don't you ever feel... isolated? Being so far from family and friends, doesn't the homesickness weigh on you?"

Her breath hitched, the question catching her off guard. No one had ever asked her that so plainly. For a moment, her composure wavered, and a flicker of something raw crossed her face. She looked at him, her voice quieter, almost confessional.

"Shamik, you can't imagine how much it does. This job—it's a world of its own, full of new places and people. But it takes so much from you. Four to six months at a time, you're gone, missing weddings, birthdays, the moments that matter. You try to stay connected, but the internet is slow, expensive, and you're too tired to keep up. Your family becomes distant, like you're slipping out of their lives. Friends move on, and you're left trying to explain this strange existence to people who can't understand. I regret it, sometimes taking this path. If you have family, do a year, perhaps two, then return to them. Don't let this life steal those bonds. You'll meet remarkable people, maybe even find love, but the cost… it's heavy."

Shamik stood still, her words settling over him like a tide. The ship's low hum filled the silence.

Leana straightened, her professionalism returning, though her eyes held a trace of vulnerability. "I've said enough. Get yourself ready and meet me at the medical centre in twenty minutes. We have work to do."

She turned and left, her footsteps echoing faintly as Shamik watched her go, the gravity of her words lingering in the small cabin.

Leana's footsteps echoed softly in the narrow corridor as she walked away from Shamik's cabin, the hum of the ship a constant undertone. Her chest felt tight, as if her words to him had unlocked something she'd kept buried for too long. Why had she said that? She was meant to inspire new nurses, to guide them through the chaos of this floating world, to train them to thrive. Yet, instead, she'd poured out her regrets, warning him to flee this life before it claimed him. She couldn't fathom what had compelled her to be so unguarded.

Her mind drifted, unbidden, to memories she rarely allowed herself to touch. She thought of David, her ex-husband, his face once so familiar but now blurred by time. When he'd lost his job, the weight of their debts—his reckless spending, her own student loans—had crushed them both. This job, with its promise of steady pay and distance from their crumbling life, had seemed like salvation. She'd signed on as a cruise ship nurse, thinking the money would mend their fractures, that it would buy them time to rebuild. But it hadn't.

She'd wanted children, had dreamt of in vitro, of building a family to fill the quiet spaces in her heart. But David had betrayed her, his infidelity a wound that cut deeper than she'd ever admitted. The divorce had left her untethered, and the ship had become her refuge—a place to outrun the pain. Yet, even here, loneliness followed her like a shadow.

Leana paused at a porthole, the sea stretching endlessly beyond, its surface deceptively calm. She'd tried to find connection on these ships, had let herself believe in the spark of new relationships. There had been men—charming, fleeting presences who spoke of adventure and shared late-night confidences in the crew mess. But too often, their promises unravelled. Some were married, their vows hidden behind easy smiles; others vanished when their contracts ended, leaving her with nothing but echoes of what might have been. Each time, she'd felt the ache of isolation grow sharper, a reminder that this life, for all its bustle, could be profoundly solitary.

Perhaps Shamik's question had stirred it all up—his innocent query about homesickness piercing a truth she'd avoided. She had no family waiting for her, no children to anchor her, no friends close enough to bridge the gap of months at sea. The ship was her world, but it was a transient one, where bonds formed quickly and broke just as fast. Maybe she'd warned him because she wished someone had warned her, years ago, before this life became her only home.

She pressed a hand to her forehead, exhaling slowly. She couldn't keep carrying this alone—the weight of her choices, the longing for something more. Perhaps it was time to speak to someone, to unravel the tangle of her thoughts with a counsellor, someone who could help her make sense of it all. The ship had resources, she knew, though she'd always shied away, too proud to admit she needed help. But pride hadn't eased the emptiness.

With a final glance at the sea, Leana straightened, her resolve firming. She'd train Shamik, do her job, keep the medical centre running. But she'd also take that first step—find someone to talk to, to help her find a path forward. For now, though, there was work to be done. She turned and continued down the corridor, the hum of the ship steady beneath her feet, carrying her into the next moment.

Shamik stepped into the medical centre, his crisp scrubs marking him as ready for the challenges ahead. "I'm here, Leana," he said, his voice steady but tinged with nervous anticipation.

Leana glanced up from her clipboard, offering a brief nod. "Good. Let's get started." She led him through the compact facility, its sterile walls lined with neatly organised supplies and equipment. As she explained the layout—examination rooms, emergency kits, the defibrillator's location—Shamik scribbled notes with fierce concentration, his pen moving almost as fast as her words.

"This first week is intensive," Leana said, pausing by the medication cabinet. "You'll have training sessions daily—protocols, passenger care, emergency drills. By next week, you'll be taking calls on your own, so focus now. It's a steep learning curve."

Shamik nodded, his expression resolute, though his hand faltered briefly as he wrote. Leana watched him for a moment, then lowered her voice, her tone softer but firm. "One more thing, Shamik. What I said earlier, outside your cabin—it was unprofessional. I shouldn't have burdened you with my regrets. Please, keep it between us."

He looked up, setting his notebook down, his eyes meeting hers with quiet sincerity. "Leana, thank you for saying what you did. I needed to hear it. I have three children at home, a wife, and I'm here for them—to give them a better future. Your honesty… it reminds me why I must stay focused, but also why I can't let this job take everything. I'm grateful."

Leana's breath caught, his words stirring the ache she'd tried to suppress. She managed a small smile, masking the flicker of guilt for her earlier candour. "You're welcome," she said simply, then gestured to the chart on the wall. "Now, let's go over the triage procedures. We've a long shift ahead."

At 6:00 pm, the entire medical team gathered in the meeting room, the ship's low hum a steady pulse beneath their feet. Before the agenda could begin, Shamik rose, introducing himself unprompted.

"Hello, everyone. My name is Shamik, from South Africa. I worked in a government hospital's trauma and casualty unit. I am married, with three children, and my wife is a neonatal intensive care nurse. The medications and equipment here are unfamiliar to me, and I anticipate challenges. You are the only family I have on this ship, and I would greatly appreciate your support to help me achieve my goals."

Leana was taken aback by his candour, her breath catching at his call for unity. Dr. Gutierrez spoke next, his voice measured. "I am Dr. Gutierrez, and I have worked on cruise ships for the past ten years. Before that, I spent a decade in trauma care in Mexico. I am married, with two children, and I took this job because the pay is better than in my country."

Jit followed, her tone curt but clear. "I am Jit, from Thailand, single. I have been on this ship for twelve years—no boyfriend, no children, no husband."

Dr. Srinivas stood, his expression weary. "I am Srinivas, from Kerala, India. This is my first contract, and it has been challenging—the long hours, the exhaustion, my ups and downs. But, as Shamik said, we are a family, and we need each other's support."

Gutierrez and Leana exchanged a glance, a silent question lingering. During the past cruise, Srinivas's three errors—tardiness and oversights—had nearly compromised patient care. Should they overlook it, given his newness, like Shamik, or address it directly?

Mkhwanazi rose, her smile warm. "I am Mkhwanazi, from Johannesburg. I have two daughters, a husband on land, and a husband at sea."

The team erupted in laughter, the tension easing. "I have needs too," Mkhwanazi added, her eyes twinkling. "I am here to embrace life."

Finally, Roberta spoke, her voice bright. "I am Roberta, from Brazil—a model and fitness enthusiast, eager to explore the world. I worked in publishing administration before this. I love this job."

After the introductions, Gutierrez, his trauma surgeon's resolve etched deep, inspired by Shamik's words, addressed Ni Luh's case, his voice firm. "In the future, a pelvic examination is non-negotiable. Her hospitalisation was our oversight, a mistake we cannot repeat. A pelvic check might have prevented her distress, but, thankfully, her baby is safe."

Leana, moved by Shamik's emphasis on family, spoke next.
"We faced challenges on a previous cruise," she stated, her tone steady. "Jit's missed calls and Srinivas's tardiness caused issues, but we must put those behind us and learn from them."

Shamik leaned forward, his voice gentle but assured. "Let us eat together."

For the first time, the entire team walked to the mess as a unit, their dinner shared in newfound camaraderie.

Leana observed Shamik, a quiet certainty settling within her. She thought to herself, He is undoubtedly lead nurse material.

Coming soon
Voyage 002 Cruising with the New hire